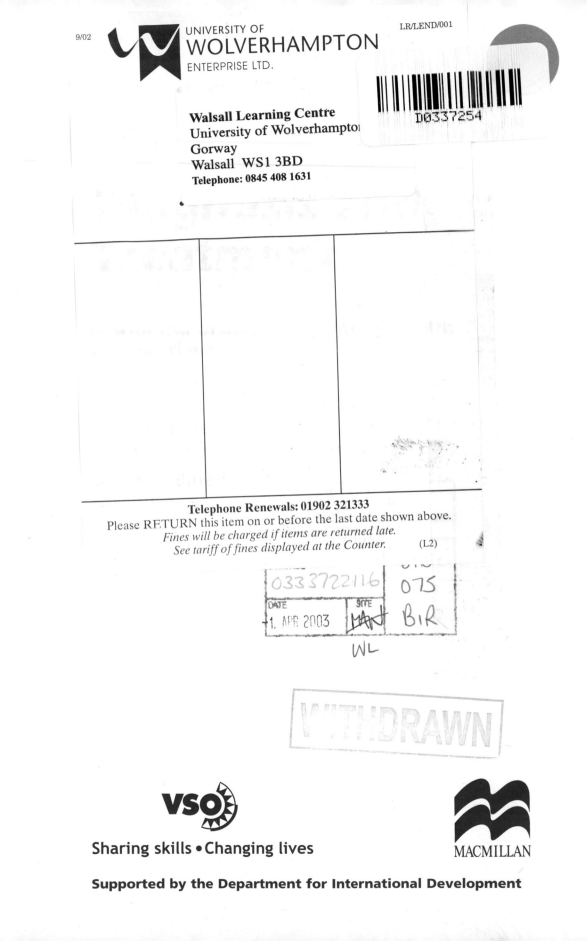

VSO

Sharing skills • Changing lives

MACMILLAN

Supported by the Department for International Development

First published 2000 by
MACMILLAN EDUCATION LTD
London and Oxford
Companies and representatives throughout the world

ISBN 0–333–72211–6

10   9   8   7   6   5   4   3   2   1
09 08 07 06 05 04 03 02 01 00

This book is printed on paper suitable for recycling and made from fully managed and sustained forest sources.

Printed in China

A catalogue record for this book is available from the British Library.

Illustrations by TechType

Cover photos are courtesy of VSO and Rob Cousins (top left), Susan Hackett (top right), Matthew Mawson (bottom right), Caroline Penn (bottom left)

Contents

Foreword by Dr Jonathan Quick, Director, EDM, WHO   v
Acknowledgements   vi

Introduction   1

Part 1   Basic skills   3

Chapter 1   How to use this manual   3
Chapter 2   How to take a patient's history   7
Chapter 3   Communication   12

Part 2   The lessons   15

Lesson 1   Rational prescribing   15
Lesson 2   Chest illnesses   25
Lesson 3   Fever, malaria, convulsions and meningitis   38
Lesson 4   Malnutrition and anaemia   51
Lesson 5   Skin problems   70
Lesson 6   Diarrhoea   85
Lesson 7   Women's health problems   95
Lesson 8   Abdominal problems   104
Lesson 9   Heart problems   124
Lesson 10   Accidents, emergencies, joints and the back   132
Lesson 11   Psychiatric problems   147
Lesson 12   Tuberculosis and leprosy   160
Lesson 13   HIV disease   169
Lesson 14   Ear, nose and throat problems   179
Lesson 15   Eye problems   189

Part 3   Appendices   205

Appendix 1   How to treat children aged 5 years or less, who have a cough or difficult breathing   206
Appendix 2   How to treat patients aged 6 years or more, who have a cough or difficult breathing   207
Appendix 3   How to give injections   208
Appendix 4   How to give diazepam rectally   210
Appendix 5   How to make a measuring bottle for liquid medicines   211
Appendix 6   How to treat malnutrition and anaemia   212
Appendix 7   How to set up a nutrition clinic   213
Appendix 8   Sickle cell disease   217

Contents

Appendix 9 How to make treatments for fungus infections 219
Appendix 10 How to treat diarrhoea 220
Appendix 11 How to put in a nasogastric tube 221
Appendix 12 Other treatments for diarrhoea 222
Appendix 13 Polio 224
Appendix 14 How to treat a woman with pain in the lower abdomen or unusual discharge from the private parts 226
Appendix 15 How to treat obstetric problems 227
Appendix 16 Diabetes 229
Appendix 17 How to interpret urine results 231
Appendix 18 How to treat a patient with abdominal pain or with blood in the faeces 232
Appendix 19 How to diagnose the cause of back pain 233
Appendix 20 How to treat an ear problem 234
Appendix 21 How to treat an eye problem 235
Appendix 22 Prescribers' checklists – trainer's copy and students' copy 237
Appendix 23 List of medicines and their uses 245

Glossary 254
List of useful resources for health workers 258
Index 260

Foreword

Nearly 54 million people died worldwide in 1998, the majority of them in developing countries. Many of these deaths were easily avoidable. Proven medicines or vaccines could have prevented millions of deaths from conditions such as pneumonia, malaria and tuberculosis. Iron-folate preparations could have prevented considerable maternal and child mortality by reducing anaemia in pregnancy. Treatment of sexually transmissible infections and use of condoms could have significantly reduced AIDS virus transmission. Treatment of hypertension could have prevented many cases of heart attack and stroke.

The drugs that could have prevented these deaths are commonly termed 'essential drugs'. Essential drugs together can provide safe, effective treatment for the majority of communicable and non-communicable diseases. But their potential can be realised only if the relevant drugs are accessible, affordable, of good quality, and used rationally. Unfortunately, irrational drug use (such as overuse of antibiotics and injections, and insufficient use of effective products) is common. It can lead to treatment failure, development of drug resistance; wastage of limited family and community resources, and drug shortages.

Understanding that much irrational drug use stems quite simply from lack of information and training, VSO has developed *Diagnosis and Treatment: A Training Manual for Primary Health Care Workers*. Based on extensive field experience and field testing, this manual will help primary health care workers use essential drugs to effectively combat the ill health that continues to hinder human well-being and development in the world's poorest countries.

Dr Jonathan D. Quick
Director,
Department of Essential Drugs and Other Medicines,
World Health Organization, Geneva

Acknowledgements

The authors wish to thank the following people. Without their help, this book would be much less helpful as a resource for trainers and students. Although every effort has been made to ensure the accuracy of the text, any errors are ours, not theirs:

Dr A.O. Adebajo, Consultant Rheumatologist, Barnsley District Hospital NHS Trust, UK; Dr Hugh Alberti, General Practitioner, Middlesbrough, UK; Penny Amerena, Head of VSO Books, London, UK; Kathy Attawell, freelance medical editor, formerly of Healthlink, London, UK; Professor A.H. Barnett, Professor of Medicine, University of Birmingham, UK; Mr Bashir Waziri Mohammed, Save the Children, Zanzibar; Silke Bernau, VSO Books Editor, London, UK; Dr Jim Birch, Consultant Psychiatrist, North Shields Community Mental Health Team, UK; Dr Luke Birmingham, Clinical Senior Lecturer in Forensic Psychology, Fareham, UK; Dr Fraser Birrell, Clinical Research Fellow, ARC Epidemiology Research Unit, University of Manchester, UK; Dr Rachel Bishop, Himalayan Trust, Khunde Hospital, The Khumbu, Nepal; Dr B. Brabin, Senior Lecturer in Tropical Paediatrics, Liverpool School of Tropical Medicine, Honorary Consultant Community Paediatrician, UK; Dr James Bunn, Lecturer in Tropical Medicine, Liverpool School of Tropical Medicine, UK; Dr Mary Bunn, General Practitioner, Liverpool, UK; Professor Nimrod Bwibo, Professor of Paediatrics, University of Nairobi, Kenya; Dr Harry Campbell, Senior Lecturer, Department of Public Health Sciences, University of Edinburgh, UK; Mr Ben Casey, Surgical Nurse, Leeds General Hospital, UK; Professor Alan Fleming, formerly Professor of Haematology at Ahmadu Bello University, University of Witwatersrand and University of Zambia; Dr Paul Garner, Senior Lecturer in Tropical Medicine, Liverpool School of Tropical Medicine, UK; Dr Charles Gilks, Senior Lecturer in Tropical Medicine, Liverpool School of Tropical Medicine, UK; Dr David Goodall, Consultant Obstetrician and Gynaecologist, Blackburn, Hyndburn and Ribble Valley Health Care Trust, UK; Dr Fiona Hampton, Consultant Paediatrician, South Cleveland General Hospital, UK; Dr A. Harley, Consultant Cardiologist, The Cardiothoracic Centre, Liverpool NHS Trust, UK; Mr C. Holcombe, Consultant Surgeon, The Royal Liverpool Hospitals, UK; Dr D.W. Jones, General Practitioner, Ryton, Northumberland, UK; Mr M.G. Kerr-Muir, Consultant Ophthalmologist, Addenbrooke's, Cambridge, UK; Associate Professor Yap Hui Kim, Professor in Paediatric Nephrology, National University Hospital Singapore; Dr Jim Litch, Himalayan Trust, Khunde Hospital, The Khumbu, Nepal; Dr Hans Martin-Hirt, Action for Nature and Medicine, Germany; Professor David Morley, Emeritus Professor of Child Health, Institute of Child Health, London, UK; Dr M.S. McCormick, Consultant ENT Surgeon, The Royal Liverpool University Hospitals, UK; Ms Nadya Haroub Nassor, Save the Children, Zanzibar, Tanzania; Dr Paul Newton, Hospital for Tropical Diseases, Mahidol University, Bangkok, Thailand; Dr John Orley, retired director of Psychiatric Division of WHO; Dr E.M.E. Poskitt, Head of Station, Dunn Nutrition Group, Keneba, Gambia; Mr Salim Hamad Ameir, Mkwajuni School, Zanzibar, Tanzania; Professor Frank Shann, Royal Children's Hospital, Parkville, Victoria, Australia; Dr Sira Ubwa Mamboya, Tuberculosis Control Programme, Zanzibar, Tanzania; Mr Dave Smith, science teacher, Parliament Hill School, London, UK; Dr B. Squire, Senior Lecturer in Tropical Medicine, Liverpool School of Tropical Medicine, UK; Georgina Stock, Editor of *Practical Pharmacy*, previously VSO pharmacist, Dareda Hospital, Tanzania; Mr Suleiman Salim Othuman, student, Potoa School, Zanzibar, Tanzania; Dr Talib Mahadhi Ali, Primary Health Care Support Programme, Zanzibar, Tanzania; Dr Martin Tobin, Lecturer in Public Health Medicine, Leicester, previously Action Health, Pemba, Tanzania; Dr Tracey Tobin,

General Practitioner Leicester, previously Action Health, Pemba, Tanzania; Dr Elizabeth Topley, retired Professor in Department of Preventive and Social Medicine, University College Hospital, Ibadan, Nigeria; Professor N.J. White, Hospital for Tropical Diseases, Mahidol University, Bangkok, Thailand; Dr Mark Woodhead, Consultant in General and Respiratory Medicine, Manchester Royal Infirmary, UK; Dr G.B. Wyatt, Senior Lecturer in Tropical Medicine, Liverpool School of Tropical Medicine, Honorary Consultant Physician, UK; Ms Zulpha Suleiman Omar, Save the Children, Zanzibar, Tanzania.

Keith Birrell and Ginny Birrell

VSO Books, the authors and the publishers are grateful to the following for permission to reproduce copyright material: TALC for Pictures 1, 8 and 9 and the growth charts used in Pictures 11, 12 and 13; WHO for Picture 3, Chest Indrawing, from *The Management of Acute Respiratory Infections in Children – Practical guidelines for outpatient care*, WHO, Geneva, 1995; Professor Emeritus David Morley for providing the growth charts and information for Pictures 5 to 7; and Dr Hans-Martin Hirt and Bindanda M'Pia for Picture 55 and the recipe for anti-fungal treatment in Appendix 9, from *Natural Medicine in the Tropics*, Hirt, H-M. and M'Pia, B., Anamed, 1995 (available from Anamed, Schafweide 77, D-71364 Winnenden, Germany). Some of the concepts of the story in Lesson 1 are very loosely based upon the slide set *Essential Drugs*, available from TALC.

This book is dedicated to our teachers and our students.
It is also dedicated to Raymond Birrell.

Introduction

Primary health care workers see patients before any other trained health workers. Primary health care workers diagnose common and important health problems and prescribe medicines. However, they may have little formal medical training and little access to help and advice. They often work in health centres with few medicines or resources. Good training for primary health care workers is, therefore, very important.

Who is this manual for?

This is a training manual for primary health care workers who work in first-level clinics, dispensaries and health centres in the developing world. Primary health care workers include nurses, medical assistants, doctors, health aides, village health workers and other paramedical health workers.

This manual will help to teach these primary health care workers how to diagnose common illnesses and how to prescribe rationally. The manual is based on a training course that was first developed in Tanzania by VSO doctors and their local colleagues. A wide range of health experts has helped to adapt that original training course to make it relevant to primary health care workers throughout the developing world.

Rational prescribing means giving the correct medicine in the correct dose for the correct length of time. It means that medicine is only prescribed if it is needed. Rational prescribing helps health workers to provide good care for their patients and to make the best use of limited supplies of medicines.

The medicines recommended in this manual are based on WHO guidelines for the use of essential drugs. The care and treatment advice in this manual is also consistent with the most important aspects of WHO's Integrated Management of Childhood Illnesses (IMCI) programme.

How can you use the manual?

The manual can be used as:
- a course guide for trainers and supervisors of primary health care workers
- a self-study guide for primary health care students.

Part 1 of the manual starts with the basic skills which health workers need for rational prescribing. Chapter 1 tells you how to use this manual. Chapter 2 explains how to take a history, and Chapter 3 discusses communication. Part 2 has 15 lessons about the most important and common health problems in developing countries. Part 3 contains 23 appendices which include reference charts, a list of medicines and their uses, and details about health problems which are only common in some areas. They provide more detailed practical information about diagnosis, treatment and procedures. Many appendices are used during the lessons.

The lessons teach primary health care workers:
- how to diagnose and treat illness
- when to send patients to hospital
- how to give advice to prevent illness.

Trainers can use the lessons as part of a training course for primary health care workers. If you are a primary health care worker or a student of primary health care, you can use the lessons to teach yourself. Whether you are a trainer or a student, you should start with Chapter 2 and Chapter 3.

If necessary, trainers and students should adapt the manual so it is consistent with the national drug policy and clinical care guidelines in your country. The advice in this manual is not intended to replace national drug and care policy. **You should adapt the course to fit guidance in your country wherever the treatment and prescribing advice in the manual is different from your national policy.**

You can change the order of the lessons and start with the most important or most common health problems in your country. The manual does not include all illnesses. You can ask a doctor or an experienced prescriber to produce extra lessons about other illnesses that are important in your country. You can also leave out parts of lessons about illnesses that are not important where you work.

Note on language

Health workers and patients are male or female. That is why, in this manual, we sometimes use 'she' when we talk about health workers and patients, and sometimes we use 'he'. We use 'mother' to describe the carer of child patients.

Girls are often at a greater disadvantage than their brothers. However, we have decided to use 'he' when we talk about child patients with their mothers, so that it is always clear that 'he' is the child, and 'she' is the child's carer.

Guidelines for trainers

Planning the course

If your trainees are already primary health care workers, plan the course over a minimum of 15 months. Teaching one lesson each month allows students to practise using new information and skills at their places of work. It also gives you a chance to observe your students at work to see how much they have learned and to help them improve.

If you are planning a course for student health workers, plan to teach one lesson each week. Teach in the language that students understand best.

Start with the lessons in Chapter 2 and 3 about taking a history and communication. Teach these chapters to each student individually. Show the student how to take a history and how to communicate. Use real patients. Allow the student to practise with patients and watch what he does. Tell the student what he has done well and show him what he can do better.

Next, start to teach the 15 lessons about common health problems. After each lesson, give students the opportunity to try out their new diagnosis and prescribing knowledge and skills with patients. At first, students will make many mistakes. Your job is to help the students to learn from their mistakes and to improve.

Before the lessons

You need to prepare posters and other teaching aids before each lesson. You may need to ask some students to help you in the lesson. We tell you at the beginning of each lesson what you need to do before the lesson. Practise what you are going to teach before the lesson.

Arrange for each student to visit a TB clinic and a leprosy clinic during the course. Give each student a copy of Table 1 in Lesson 12 before they visit the clinics. Ask TB and leprosy doctors at the clinics to show the students each of the symptoms in the table.

Planning the lessons

Each lesson in Part 2, except Lesson 1, starts with a quiz that the students do on their own. The quiz helps the students to find out what they know and what they need to learn more about. At the end of the lesson, the trainer repeats the quiz and gives the correct answers. Doing the quiz again helps the students to see how much they have learnt.

Most teaching sessions last about 5 hours, including breaks. Plan regular breaks, with refreshments, every 2 hours.

For example, if the session starts in the morning:
- Ask students to arrive at 8.30 am. Students should start by answering the quiz.
- Start the lesson at 9.00 am.
- Break at 11.00 am for 15–30 minutes for refreshments.
- Start to teach again at 11.30 am.
- Finish the lesson at 1.30 pm.

Teaching methods

We learn by hearing, seeing and doing – especially by doing. We also learn by repeating things. Remember the saying 'If I hear I forget, if I see I remember, if I do I know'.

The lessons use different teaching methods that involve hearing, seeing and doing. These methods include role plays, demonstrations, discussions and examination of patients. You do not have to use the methods suggested in the manual. The book *Helping Health Workers Learn* by David Werner and Bill Bower has many other good ideas about other teaching methods. If you try a different teaching method and it works well, please write and tell the authors: Dr Keith Birrell and Dr Ginny Birrell, c/o VSO Books, 317 Putney Bridge Road, London SW15 2PN, UK.

Encourage students to ask questions during the lesson. Make sure students are not embarrassed about giving the wrong answer. Make sure that all students are involved, not just one or two talkative ones.

How to use the posters

Before each lesson, write the number and title of each poster on a very large sheet of paper or a flipchart. The lessons use three types of poster:

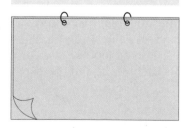

POSTER
(Prepared poster)

POSTER
(Student answer poster)

POSTER
(Summary poster)

1. **Prepared poster:** You can complete these posters before the lesson. The information for the posters is given in the text.

2. **Student answer poster:** These are posters which you complete during the lesson with the participation of students. Summarise the students' correct answers on the poster as they call them out. After the students have finished giving you their answers, tell them any answers they have missed. Add the summary words for the missing answers to the poster. You can use pencil to write the summary words of the correct answers in small letters on the poster before the lesson to remind you. The summary words you need are written in the text in **bold** or are presented in a table or box.

3. **Summary poster:** You will complete these posters yourself during the lesson as you teach. You can use pencil to write the summary words of the correct answers in small letters on the poster before the lesson to remind you. The summary words you need are written in the text in **bold**.

For example, if we ask you to summarise these sentences about feeding children:

> **Breastfeed** children **until** they reach **2 years** of age. **Never use a bottle** to feed children. Bottles are very difficult to clean. The bacteria in bottles cause diarrhoea. Diarrhoea can kill children. **Use a cup and spoon** to give fluids.

Write only the important summary words in **bold** on the poster:

> **Breastfeed until 2 years**
> **Never use a bottle**
> **Use a cup and a spoon**

Follow-up

After each lesson, the trainer must observe each student at work in her health centre or practising with patients. Repeat advice about how to diagnose and treat patients. Remind the student of what she learned in the classroom.

Use the prescriber's checklist in Appendix 22 to help you to follow up each student. Use the trainer's copy to remind you what the student was taught. Use the student's copy to write down three things she does well and three things she could do better. Discuss these things with the student. Praise her when she does something well. Show her how to improve. Tell the student that the next time you visit the health centre, you will look to see if she has improved.

If a student has problems, the trainer can role-play a patient who has an illness: tell the student what she would find if she examined such a patient. Then, help the student to ask the correct questions and to do a good examination. Ask her what illness the patient has and what the treatment is for the illness. Help her to give the correct answer. If a student is learning very slowly, there is usually a good reason. Ask her what the problem is and help her to overcome it.

Guidelines for students

If you are a health worker or a student, you can study this manual on your own and learn at your own speed. Learning will be easier if you work with an experienced prescriber. This prescriber will be your 'trainer'. Ask him to watch your work, to tell you what you do well and to correct your mistakes. You can also discuss the questions and information in the manual with other health workers and help each other to learn.

Planning your learning

The course has 15 lessons. Try to do one lesson each month. Use the new knowledge and new skills in your work after each lesson. If you do not understand something, write it down. Ask another health worker to help you and to answer your questions. Do not be afraid to admit that you do not know something.

Start by doing the quiz at the start of each lesson. The quiz will show you what you know and do not know. Do the quiz again at the end of the lesson, to see how much your knowledge has improved. Act out the demonstrations and role plays together with other students or health workers in your health centre. Discuss the examples of patients with your colleagues before looking at the answers. If you think a table or diagram is useful, draw it and put it on the wall in your health centre so you can refer to it. Before you start the next lesson, try to answer the quiz from the last lesson. If many of your answers are not correct, perhaps you need to read that lesson again.

Chapter 2 How to take a patient's history

BEFORE THE LESSON

- Remember to teach each student individually to make sure that each student understands this important subject.

- Give each student a copy of this chapter to read before the lesson.

- Give each student a copy of Appendix 4.

- If there is no malaria in your area, cross out the box in this lesson about malaria treatment.

Start by explaining the information below to the student. Then, see patients together with each student. Show the student how to take a patient's history. Ask the student to practise talking to patients while you watch. Tell the student what he does correctly. Show the student how to improve. Do not expect the student to understand all the answers that the patient gives. Tell the student what the diagnosis is and how to treat the patient.

You do not have much time with each patient. Sometimes you may have less than 5 minutes to decide what illness the patient has and what treatment to prescribe. In this time, you must also give the patient advice to help her to use her medicine correctly and to help her stay healthy.

To diagnose and treat patients you need to:
1. ask the patient the correct questions
2. examine the correct parts of the patient
3. make sure that the patient will use the medicine correctly and follow your advice.

This lesson teaches you how to ask the right questions. This is called taking a history. Before you learn how to take a history, you need to know about general danger signs and how to treat very severe febrile disease.

General danger signs

There are four general danger signs:
1. The patient is unconscious or moves less than usual when he is awake.
2. The patient has had a convulsion (also called a fit).
3. The patient has vomited four times or more this morning.
4. The patient is not able to drink or breastfeed.

A patient with any of these four general danger signs may be very ill. He may have severe malaria, pneumonia or meningitis. Severe malaria, pneumonia and meningitis are very severe febrile diseases.

If a patient has a general danger sign, you do not need to take a full history. Treat him immediately for a very severe febrile disease and send him straight to hospital.

Treatment for very severe febrile diseases

1. If the patient has vomited, clear his mouth with your finger. Lay him on his side.
2. If the patient has fever, take him to a warm room and remove his clothes. Wipe him with a warm, wet cloth to cool him. This is called tepid sponging.
3. If the patient is having a convulsion, give him diazepam rectally (see Appendix 4). Repeat the dose of diazepam if the patient is still having a convulsion 5 minutes after taking the first dose. Diazepam dosages are shown in Table 1.

TABLE 1 Doses of diazepam

Age	Dose
Up to 1 year	2.5 mg
1–3 years	5 mg
3 years or more	10 mg

4. To prevent low blood sugar:
   - If the patient can breastfeed, ask the mother to breastfeed.
   - If the patient is not able to breastfeed but can drink, use a cup and spoon to give him expressed breastmilk, or a breastmilk substitute or sugar water. Give 30–50 ml of milk or sugar water. To make sugar water, mix four level teaspoons (20 g) of sugar with a cup (200 ml) of clean water.
   - If the patient is unable to drink, and you know how to use a nasogastric tube, give 50 ml of milk or sugar water by nasogastric tube.
5. Give the patient an injection of quinine intramuscularly (10 mg for each kg of body weight). Inject half the quinine into the front of each leg. If there is no quinine, give chloroquine intramuscularly (3.5 mg for each kg of body weight).
6. If the patient is NOT pregnant, NOT breast feeding or NOT less than 1 month old, give an injection of chloramphenicol intramuscularly, 40 mg or 0.2 ml for each kg of body weight. Do not give more than 1000 mg (5.6 ml) of chloramphenicol.
   - If there is no chloramphenicol, or if the patient is pregnant, breastfeeding or less than 1 month old, give benzylpenicillin intramuscularly (one dose of 0.1 million IU for each kg of body weight or 60 mg for each kg of body weight, **or** give this

dose four times a day if the patient is not able to get to the hospital immediately). Do not give more than 2 million IU of benzylpenicillin in each dose.
- If there is no benzylpenicillin, give procaine penicillin fortified (0.1 million IU for each kg of body weight or 100 mg for each kg of body weight). Do not give more than 1.2 million IU in each dose.

7. After initial treatment, send the patient to hospital immediately. Carry him flat so that his head is at the same level as his legs. Write down what treatment you have given the patient on his record card.

Taking a history

There are six important steps in taking a history. If the patient answers 'Yes' to any of the questions, you need to ask more questions after you have finished taking the history. The boxes tell you what extra questions you need to ask, or which Lesson or Appendix will tell you more about the illness.

The six steps are:

1. **Greet the patient**.

2. **Ask the patient what she thinks her problem is**.
This will normally take less than 30 seconds. Do not interrupt her until she has talked for about one minute.

> If the patient has pain in the abdomen or blood in the faeces, she may have an abdominal problem. Ask the more detailed questions in step 3, then follow the instructions for diagnosing and treating abdominal problems in Appendix 18.

If the patient has an obvious common or important problem, ask the more detailed questions in step 3, then follow the advice given in the appropriate lesson.

Finally, for all patients do steps 4, 5 and 6.

3. **Ask the patient more detailed questions about her symptoms**.
   - When did your symptoms start?
   - Have you had a fever?

> You will learn about fever in Lesson 3.

   - Have you had any convulsions? (Convulsions are also called fits.)

Convulsions are a general danger sign. Treat the patient for very severe febrile disease and send her to hospital immediately. You will learn about convulsions in Lesson 3.

- Do you have a cough? Do you have difficult breathing?

If the patient has cough or difficult breathing, follow the instructions in Appendix 1 or Appendix 2. You will learn about cough and difficult breathing in Lesson 2.

- Do you have problems with eating or drinking? Have you vomited?

If the patient is not able to eat or drink, she may be very ill. This is a general danger sign. Treat the patient for very severe febrile disease and send her to hospital immediately.

If the patient has vomited, ask her how many times she has vomited that morning. If the patient has vomited two or three times, treat her for her illness at the health centre and ask her to wait for 30 minutes. This is so you can make sure that she does not vomit up the medicine you have given her. If the patient has vomited four times or more that morning, treat her for a very severe febrile disease.

- Do you have diarrhoea? Do you have blood in your faeces?

If the patient has diarrhoea or blood in her faeces, follow the instructions for treating diarrhoea in Appendix 10 and for treating a patient with blood in the faeces in Appendix 18. You will learn about diarrhoea in Lesson 6 and about abdominal problems in Lesson 8.

- What medicines have you used in the last 2 weeks?

This question is very important if you think the patient may have malaria. To decide about treatment for malaria, you need to know if the patient has taken any malaria medicines already.

4. **Examine the patient**.
Feel the patient's forehead for a fever. Look for anaemia on the inside of the patient's lower eyelid.

5. **Check the growth chart** if the patient is a child aged 5 years or less. Make sure young children have had all their **vaccinations**.

6. **Write up your notes**. Summarise what you have found. This will help you to decide what is wrong with the patient and how to treat her.

   For example:
   Name and age: Chandan Patel, age 4 years
   History: Fever for 3 days, vomited one time
   Examination: Fever, pale, no fast breathing, growing well
   Diagnosis: Malaria and anaemia

If you do not know what the diagnosis is:
- send the patient to hospital if she is very ill
- ask the patient to come back on another day if she is not very ill.

You will learn how to make sure that the patient takes the medicine correctly and follows your advice in the next chapter.

Chapter 3   Communication

BEFORE THE LESSON

■ Remember to teach each student individually to make sure each student understands this important subject.

■ Give each student a copy of this chapter and ask them to read it before the lesson.

Start by explaining the information below to the student. Then, see patients together with each student. Show the student how to communicate with patients. Ask the student to practise talking to patients while you watch. Tell the student what she does correctly. Show her how to improve. Tell the student what the diagnosis is and how to treat the patient. Make sure that the student follows the seven rules of communication.

Primary health care workers can only help patients to get better and to stay well if they can communicate.

The health worker must be able to communicate with a patient so that:
• the patient can explain what is wrong
• the patient understands the questions the health worker is asking him and the health worker can learn what the problem is
• the patient understands what his illness is and what caused it
• the patient knows how to use his medicine correctly and how to stay well.

To be a good communicator, a health worker needs to ask questions and to listen carefully. He must also use simple language and explain things clearly. Avoid giving too much information at once. Check that the patient understands your advice.

To help you remember, use the seven rules of good communication each time you see a patient:

1. **Respect privacy**
   See patients in a quiet, private place. Patients find it easier to talk if they are not worried about someone else listening to what they say. This helps the patient to give you better information so you can make a better diagnosis. It also helps the patient to understand what you tell him about the treatment.

2. **Use simple language**
   You should use simple, clear language that the patient understands. Use local words and avoid medical terms. If the

patient does not understand, he may become confused or may not follow your advice.

3. Give enough time

Give the patient enough time to explain his problems. If you do not give enough time to hear the patient's history, you will not know what is wrong or how to treat him. If you do not listen, the patient may ignore your advice.

4. Show interest

Show the patient that you are interested in his problem. If the patient thinks that you are interested, he is more likely to trust your advice. Use ways of showing interest that are acceptable in your culture. For example, sit close to the patient and look at him while you are speaking. Do **not** sit on the other side of a table from him.

5. Explain

Explain to the patient what you think the problem is. Explain the treatment. Tell him how long it will take to get well. Explain when he should come back to the health centre.

6. Give one medicine

Explain to the patient how to take the medicine. Try to only give the patient one medicine. If a patient has too many medicines to take, he may forget your advice or get confused. If the patient does not need any medicine, tell him why (see also Rational Prescribing in Lesson 1). If the patient has more than one illness, treat the most important illness first. Explain to the patient that he needs to come back for treatment for his other illnesses.

7. Check understanding

Make sure that the patient fully understands his illness and the treatment. Ask the patient to repeat what you have told him. Correct anything which he has not understood correctly.

BEFORE THE LESSON

- There are three posters in this lesson. (See p. 4 for information on how to use the posters.)
  Prepared poster: 2
  Student answer posters: 1 and 3

- Give each student a pen and a notebook.

- Choose five students to help you with the demonstrations. Give them copies of the demonstrations and practise with them before the lesson.

- Give each student a copy of Chapter 3.

- Prepare one copy of the questions for the practical activity in section 3 for every five students. If you have 20 students, you will need four copies of the questions.

- Give each student a copy of Appendix 23.

Start by reading the story in section 1 to the students. (Some of the concepts of this story are very loosely based upon *Essential Drugs*, a slide set available from TALC, see List of useful resources, p. 258.)

SECTION 1:   A story

This is a story about Baki, the health assistant in the village of Bilaelimu. Baki has never been trained to diagnose and treat illnesses, but he lives in the village and cares about the health of its people. Baki's story and the story of some of his patients will teach you how to choose the correct medicine for your patients and how to avoid wasting medicines, by prescribing rationally.

First patient

Baki's first patient is Mkulima, a 24-year-old farmer. Mkulima had a cough, but was unable to go to the health centre because he had to plant his fields. He asked his friend to buy him some antibiotics from a shopkeeper.

Ask your students: What are the problems of buying medicines from a shop? Look for the following answers:

Answer   No diagnosis is made, so the patient may be treated for the wrong illness. No advice is given about how to take the medicine.

Answer   The patient receives the wrong medicine.

Answer   The wrong dose of medicine is used.

Answer   The patient uses the medicine for the wrong length of time.

Mkulima had an upper respiratory infection. Upper respiratory infections are usually caused by viruses and get better without medicine. However, the shopkeeper gave Mkulima an antibiotic called co-trimoxazole. Antibiotics are *only* used to treat illnesses caused by bacteria.

Co-trimoxazole can sometimes cause side effects, including a painful mouth and eyes. (Side effects are unwanted effects caused by medicines.) Unfortunately, this happened to Mkulima after he had taken the medicine for 2 days. He should stop taking the medicine.

Ask your students: What medicines can cause side effects? Which side effects have you seen or heard of? Look for the following answers:

Answer   Antibiotics are commonly used medicines that can cause side effects. These side effects include skin rashes, diarrhoea and nausea.

Answer   All medicines sometimes cause side effects. Only give a medicine if it is more likely to help the patient than to harm him.

POSTER 1:
(Student answer poster)

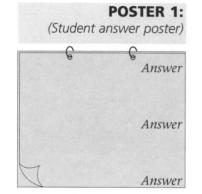

Answer

Answer

Answer

Second patient

Patient advice

Ask the students: What advice can you give a patient so that he will be happy if you do not give him medicines?

Teach the patient **about** his **illness**. Tell him that he will get better without using medicine. Tell him that using the **wrong medicine may make** him very **ill**. The wrong medicine may kill him.

Give advice to encourage healthy practices: eat a **mixed diet**, drink **clean water and wash hands** after going to the toilet and before preparing food.

Tell him how to avoid catching infectious diseases.

A mother brings her 11-month-old son, Surua, to see Baki. Surua has had a cough and fever for 5 days. Baki notices a slightly raised rash on Surua's face and neck. Surua's mother tells Baki that this rash appeared yesterday.

Show the students the picture of a child with measles (Picture 1).

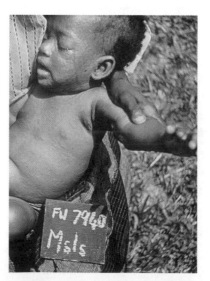

PICTURE 1   *A child with measles*

Baki asks Surua's mother questions to check for general danger signs. He finds out that Surua has had no convulsions, has not vomited and is able to feed a little. Surua has passed loose faeces three times this morning, but there is no blood in the faeces. Surua has not had any medicine in the last 2 weeks.

Next, Baki examines Surua. He finds that Surua has a fever, but is not anaemic or dehydrated and does not have pneumonia. He notices that Surua has conjunctivitis (an eye infection). Baki cannot test for malaria.

Baki decides that Surua has measles. Unfortunately, Baki does not know about rational prescribing.

He decides to give Surua:
1. co-trimoxazole to try to prevent pneumonia
2. tetracycline eye ointment to treat the conjunctivitis
3. paracetamol to treat the fever
4. first-line malaria treatment, in case the fever is caused by malaria. Malaria is common in Bilaelima.

Ask your students: Can you remember the treatments Baki gave to Surua? What do you think about the treatment that Baki gave? Look for the following answers:

Answer   Baki gave Surua four different medicines. Surua's mother may not remember how to give Surua all the medicines correctly.

Answer   Baki gave Surua three medicines that he does not need. This is wasteful because it means that Baki will not be able to give these medicines to other patients who may need them.

Before Surua and his mother leave the health centre, Baki's new trainer, Mzee, arrives. Mzee is teaching Baki about rational prescribing. He tells Baki what he has done well. Baki has taken a good history, done a good examination and decided on the correct diagnosis of measles and possible malaria. Mzee tells Baki that only two medicines will help Surua get better.

Ask the students to tell you which two medicines are most important for Surua. Help them to give you the following answers:

Answer   **First-line malaria treatment**
Surua has fever. He may have malaria. Surua needs the first-line malaria treatment because Baki cannot test for malaria.

Answer   **Vitamin A**
Vitamin A helps to prevent eye problems and blindness. Patients with measles need extra vitamin A.

Explain to the students why the other medicines are not needed:

Answer   **Co-trimoxazole:** patients with measles do sometimes get pneumonia. Antibiotics such as co-trimoxazole can *treat* pneumonia but *will not prevent* pneumonia. Surua does not have pneumonia so he does not need co-trimoxazole.

17

Answer **Tetracycline eye ointment:** measles causes conjunctivitis. But measles is a virus, and tetracycline eye ointment will not cure conjunctivitis if it is caused by a virus.

Answer **Paracetamol:** paracetamol is used to treat the *symptoms* of an illness, such as fever, *not the cause* of an illness. Paracetamol can help to reduce fever, but it will not help an illness get better.

Ask the students: What advice can you give to Surua's mother about preventing illness and keeping Surua well? Look for the following answers:

Answer Feeding can help a child to get better more quickly and to stay well. Advise Surua's mother to continue to breastfeed him. Advise her to give him small amounts of a mixed diet five times a day until he is well and for a week after he gets better.

Answer Advise her to mash Surua's food. Sick children find it easier to eat if their food is mashed.

Mzee explains to Baki the difference between symptomatic medicines and curative medicines:

- Symptomatic medicines are used to treat symptoms. For example, paracetamol and aspirin are used to reduce pain or fever.
- Curative medicines are used to cure an illness. For example, vitamin A cures vitamin A deficiency. Chloroquine and quinine are examples of medicines that cure malaria.

Mzee is still worried about giving Surua's mother two medicines to use at home. The mother may become confused about how to give each medicine. Mzee advises Baki that he should only give more than one medicine for the patient to take at home if he is sure that the patient knows how to take both medicines.

Mzee and Baki agree to give Surua the first-line malaria treatment and vitamin A. The dose of malaria treatment depends on which drug is used (the national drug policy in each country gives guidelines on first-line malaria treatment). Vitamin A is usually given in three doses, one at the health centre, one the next day and one on day 14. Baki will give Surua the first dose of a malaria treatment and the first dose of vitamin A before he leaves the health centre.

Mzee asks Baki what advice he can give Surua's mother to prevent convulsions. Baki tells him about tepid sponging for fever.

Ask the students to tell you what tepid sponging is. Look for the following answers:

Answer To tepid sponge: The mother takes the child to a warm room and removes the child's clothes. She puts a cloth in some slightly warm water and wipes the child's whole body so that it is wet.

She repeats this until the fever has gone. This will take less than 30 minutes.

Answer   Tepid sponging can prevent a child from having convulsions and it can make a child with a fever feel better. A child who feels better will be more likely to eat or breastfeed.

Demonstrations: Mzee teaches Baki about rational prescribing

Ask one student to play the part of Baki. You will play the part of his trainer Mzee. Baki and Mzee sit together by a table. Ask four other students to play the two patients and the patients' mothers. Practise the demonstration before the lesson. The role-players should say their lines slowly in a loud voice so that the other students can hear.

A woman comes in with an 18-month-old girl.

Third patient

Baki:	*Good morning.*
Mother:	Good morning.
Baki:	*Please take a seat.*
Mother:	Thank you.
Baki:	*Who is ill today?*
Mother:	My child Mapafu.
Baki:	*How old is she?*
Mother:	18 months.
Baki:	*What is wrong with her?*
Mother:	She has had a cough and a fever for 3 days.
Baki:	*Has she had a convulsion?*
Mother:	No.
Baki:	*Is she having problems feeding well or drinking well?*
Mother:	Yes. She is not feeding well.
Baki:	*Has she vomited?*
Mother:	No.
Baki:	*Does she have diarrhoea?*
Mother:	No.
Baki:	*What medicines have you used in the last 2 weeks?*
Mother:	Only traditional medicine.
Baki:	*Has she had all her vaccinations?*
Mother:	Yes.
Baki:	*May I see her growth chart?*
Mother:	Here it is.

Baki looks at the growth chart.

Baki: *The growth chart shows that Mapafu is growing well.*

Mzee now examines Mapafu as he talks to Baki.

Mzee: Mapafu does not have any general danger signs. There is no chest indrawing. She breathes more than 40 times in one minute, but there is no noise when she breathes in and out. Mapafu has a fever. She is not anaemic. Because she has fast breathing, we will treat her for pneumonia. Because she has a fever and we cannot test for malaria, we must treat her for malaria.

Baki writes a summary of what they have found on the chalkboard:

Name and age: Mapafu, 18 months
History: Fever and cough for 3 days
Examination: Fever, more than 40 breaths in one minute
Diagnosis: Pneumonia and possible malaria.

Mzee: You are very good at taking a history. What treatment are you going to use?
Baki: *I am going to treat Mapafu with Septrin.*
Mzee: The real name for Septrin is co-trimoxazole. Co-trimoxazole will treat pneumonia. Co-trimoxazole is also a treatment for possible malaria. However, I am worried that you call co-trimoxazole by its brand name Septrin. What happens at the end of the month after you have no co-trimoxazole left?
Baki: *If I have no more medicine, I tell patients what medicine they need to buy.*
Mzee: Co-trimoxazole is the same medicine as Septrin. Septrin is the manufacturer's name or **brand** name for the medicine. Co-trimoxazole is the medicine's real or **generic** name. Septrin is much more expensive than co-trimoxazole. When you prescribe or advise people to buy medicines, you should always use the medicine's generic name and not the brand name.
Baki: *So, I will treat Mapafu with co-trimoxazole, not Septrin.*
Mzee: Very good. That's right.

Ask the students to suggest other brand name medicines. Here are some examples of possible answers:

Answer Panadol is a brand name for the generic medicine paracetamol. Panadol costs about two times as much to buy as paracetamol.

Answer Brufen is the brand name for the generic medicine ibuprofen. Brufen costs more than two times as much as ibuprofen.

A mother and her 8-year-old boy come into the room.

Fourth patient

Baki: *Good morning.*
Mother: Good morning.
Baki: *Please take a seat.*
Mother: Thank you.
Baki: *Who is ill today?*
Mother: My child Upele.

Baki:	*How old is he?*
Mother:	8 years.
Baki:	*What is wrong with him?*
Mother:	He has a problem with his skin.
Baki:	*When did this problem start?*
Mother:	Two months ago.
Baki:	*Does he have a fever?*
Mother:	No.
Baki:	*Has he had a convulsion?*
Mother:	No.
Baki:	*Does he have a cough? Does he have difficult breathing?*
Mother:	No.
Baki:	*Is he having problems feeding well? Is he having problems drinking?*
Mother:	No
Baki:	*Does he have diarrhoea?*
Mother:	No.
Baki:	*What medicines has he used in the last 2 weeks?*
Mother:	None.

Baki examines Upele as he talks to Mzee.

Baki: Upele does not have a fever. He is not pale. I think he has scabies.

Baki writes a summary of what he has found on the chalk board:

Name and age: Upele, 8 years
History: Rash for 2 months
Examination: Scaly wrists and between fingers
Diagnosis: Scabies

Mzee:	What is the treatment for scabies?
Baki:	*A course of injections of procaine penicillin fortified.*
Mzee:	I agree that Upele has scabies. However, **injections and antibiotics are the wrong treatment for scabies.** Antibiotics treat infections caused by bacteria. But scabies is caused by a very small insect that lives under the skin. You should:

- Treat the patient for scabies with benzyl benzoate emulsion.
- If the skin is ulcerated or hot, there is also a bacterial infection. Paint the skin with gentian violet every day for 5 days before giving benzyl benzoate emulsion.
- If a very large area of skin is infected or if the skin is painful when pressed, give the patient a course of co-trimoxazole before giving benzyl benzoate emulsion.

Can you tell me why injections can be dangerous, Baki?

Baki:	*I've seen quite a few patients with big abscesses that are very difficult to treat.*
Mzee:	Injections can cause abscesses. Needles that have not been properly sterilised can also give patients serious illnesses like tetanus, HIV or hepatitis. Tablets are much safer than injections.

Baki: Doctor Mzee, can I ask you what 'rational prescribing' means?

Mzee: Excellent question! Rational prescribing is what we have been talking about today. It means only prescribing medicine when medicine is needed. It also means giving patients the correct dose of medicine for the correct length of time.

Baki: So, rational prescribing is giving patients the correct medicine, in the correct dose for the correct length of time, but only if patients need a medicine.

Mzee: Correct. Can you tell me three ways to make buying medicines cheaper?

Baki: The first way is to only give patients one medicine. The second is to use the generic medicine instead of a brand name medicine. I am not sure about the third.

Mzee: The third way is to only give patients medicines which cure illnesses rather than symptomatic medicines, which only help them feel better. Remember, Baki: Each time you prescribe a medicine for a patient, you should ask yourself:

- Does the patient need this medicine?
- Is the dose of the medicine correct?

Tell your students:

If you do not know the correct dose of the medicine, *do not guess.* Look up the correct dose in the list of medicines and their uses in Appendix 23.

Give each student a copy of Appendix 23.

Refreshment break

SECTION 2: Do patients take their medicine?

Discussion

This discussion will help students to think about what patients need to know about their treatment and medicine. Ask the students to tell you what they would do in the following examples.

DISCUSSION 1:

You are a 60-year-old man. The doctor has sent you to collect your medicine from the pharmacy. The pharmacy has a small window. It is very noisy in the pharmacy and your hearing is not very good. You cannot hear what the person behind the window is saying. The health worker gives you ten white tablets. What will you do with the medicine after you get home?

Look for the following answers:

Answer You may take the tablets in the way that you think is correct. You may not take the tablets at all because you do not know how many tablets to take or when to take them.

Answer After you feel better, you may stop taking the medicine. Because of this the illness may come back.

The person who gives out medicines must make sure that patients understand how to use their medicines.

POSTER 2:
(Prepared poster)

What to tell patients

> Tell the patient:
> - what his illness is
> - how to take his medicine at home
> - when to come back to the health centre.

Ask the patient to repeat what you have told him. Make sure he understands and correct anything he has not understood.

DISCUSSION 2:

You are a 26-year-old mother of five children. Your daughter, who is 4 years old, has pneumonia. The doctor took a history from you and examined your daughter. He told you she has a chest infection. The doctor has given you one medicine. The doctor's assistant tells you to give the girl one tablet three times a day until all the tablets are finished. He also asks you to bring the girl back after 2 days. You said that you would give your daughter all the medicine. You give the medicine correctly for 2 days and your daughter starts to feel better. You do not have time to take her back to the clinic.

POSTER 3:
(Student answer poster)

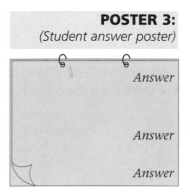

Answer

Answer

Answer

Reasons why patients take their medicine correctly

Ask the students: Will you continue to give her the medicine? Why will you?

You will give her the medicine because the **doctor listened** to what you said about your daughter. You **believe** what the **doctor** said. You believe that the **treatment** will work.

You understood that it is important to **finish all the medicine** even if the girl feels better.

The doctor and the doctor's assistant are good communicators.

SECTION 3: Practical – Deciding on the best treatment for patients

This practical activity helps students to decide on the correct treatment for patients, using the examples below. Ask the students to form small groups of five or six. Give each group a copy of what Baki and Mzee found out about three patients.

Activity

Ask each group to discuss each patient and to:

- talk about why Baki and Mzee have decided on the diagnosis for each patient
- decide if a patient needs a medicine

23

- decide what medicine to give, the correct dose and the correct length of time
- decide what advice to give the patient.

Give the students 20 minutes to do this activity.

Patient 1

The first patient is a boy aged 2 years who has fever and cough. He boy looks quite well. He breathes 30 times in one minute. He makes no noise when he breathes in and out. He weighs 12 kg.

Diagnosis: Baki and Mzee decide that he has an upper respiratory infection and possible malaria.

Patient 2

The second patient is a 6-year-old boy who has had diarrhoea for 3 days. He is still able to eat. There is no blood in his faeces. He has no fever. He is not dehydrated.

Diagnosis: Baki and Mzee decide that he has gastroenteritis.

Patient 3

The third patient is a 4-month-old boy who has had a fever since yesterday. Today he had one convulsion that lasted for 15 minutes. He has a high fever and looks ill.

Diagnosis: He has a general danger sign. Baki and Mzee decide that he has a very severe febrile disease, possibly meningitis or cerebral malaria.

Answers

Ask each group of students to give their answers. Praise the students if their answer is a correct treatment that is rational and cheap. If their answers are not correct, tell them what the best answer is and why.

Patient 1

Give him the first-line malaria treatment. Teach the mother how to reduce the fever by tepid sponging. She should bring him back to the health centre if he becomes more ill.

Patient 2

Advise the mother to give him plenty of fluids and a mixed diet. He should eat five times a day until he is better and for one week after he is better. She should bring him back to the health centre if he becomes more ill or develops a fever.

Patient 3

The mother should remove the child's clothes and treat the fever by tepid sponging. Give the child 30–50 ml of milk or sugar water to prevent low blood sugar. Give him an injection of quinine or chloroquine intramuscularly (in malaria areas), and an intramuscular injection of chloramphenicol or benzylpenicillin. Next, send him to hospital.

Ask each group to present their answers. The class can discuss the answers. Explain the correct answers.

Chest illnesses

BEFORE THE LESSON

- There are seven posters in this lesson. (See p. 4 for information on how to use the posters.)
  Prepared posters: 1, 2, 3 and 4
  Student answer posters 5, 6 and 7.
- Give each student a copy of Appendix 1, Appendix 2 and Appendix 3.
- Ask three students to act out the demonstration in the section 'Children aged 5 years or less'. Practise with them before the lesson.
- Ask two students to act out the demonstration in the section 'Adult or a child aged 6 years old or more'. Practise with them before the lesson.
- Give each student a copy of Tables 3, 4, 5 and 6.
- Bring a metered-dose inhaler of salbutamol if possible. Also bring a 1-litre plastic bottle and a knife so that you can make a spacer.
- You need to find seven patients with whom the students can practise in section 4. If possible, teach section 4 in a hospital. You can ask patients you have seen in the week before the lesson to come to the class. Patients are often willing to help new doctors to learn. Find three children aged 5 years or less: one with an upper respiratory infection, one with pneumonia and one with asthma (if possible). Also find four adults or children aged 6 years or more: one with an upper respiratory infection, one with bronchitis, one with pneumonia, and one with asthma (if possible).
- Ask the patients to arrive at 11.00 a.m. Section 4 starts after refreshments at about 11.30 a.m. Tell the patients that they will receive a small payment for coming. Do not forget to bring some money to the lesson.
- You need to ask six students to help you before the lesson and in the practical in section 4. For each of the seven patients you have asked to come to the lesson: write on a piece of paper a list of the symptoms, signs, diagnosis and treatment. Write one piece of paper for each patient. Give one piece of paper to each student and discuss it with them. You can use Appendices 1 and 2 to decide what the diagnosis is and what treatment to give each patient.

SECTION 1: Quiz

POSTER 1:
(Prepared poster)

Quiz

Ask the students to answer the questions on their own. Do not give the answers until the end of the lesson.

1. A patient who is ill may breathe fast. How many breaths in 1 minute is fast breathing:
   - for a child under the age of 2 months?

(continued)
- for a child over 2 months but under a year of age?
- for a child over a year but under 5 years of age?
- for a child 6 years or more but under 12 years of age?
- for an adult?

2. What would make you think that a patient has a severe illness which may be pneumonia or asthma?

3. Patients who find it very difficult to breathe have respiratory distress. What would you expect to see when you look at a patient with respiratory distress?

4. A patient has a cough. She is eating well. She does not have chest indrawing or fast breathing. There is no noise when she breathes in or out. She has a fever. When she coughs there is no pain in the side of her chest. She is not anaemic.
   - What illness(es) does she have?
   - What treatment should you give her?

SECTION 2: Diagnosis and management

In this section, you provide information about chest illnesses and how to diagnose and treat them.

POSTER 2:
(Prepared poster)

Bronchi and alveoli
Copy Picture 2 onto Poster 2.

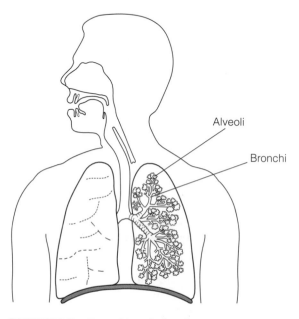

PICTURE 2 *Bronchi and alveoli*

Show the students a picture of the bronchi and alveoli and explain:

Two important things in our lungs must work so that we do not die:
- **Bronchi** – Air must be able to pass down the tubes in our lungs to reach the alveoli. These tubes are called bronchi.
- **Alveoli** – The air in the alveoli must mix with blood. Alveoli are very small pockets or sacs at the end of each tube.

Chest illnesses

1. Pneumonia

Pneumonia causes the alveoli to fill with fluid. If many alveoli fill with fluid, **the patient may die**. Pneumonia is usually caused by a bacterial infection. The patient has one, or all, of these symptoms: fever, cough, pain in his ribs when he coughs, and difficult breathing.

2. Asthma

Asthma causes the bronchi to become narrow, so air cannot get into the lung easily. The patient has difficult breathing.
If the bronchi become very narrow, the patient may die.
A patient with difficult breathing caused by asthma may make a noise when he breathes out. This is called a wheeze. It takes longer to breathe out than to breathe in. People with asthma have wheeze or difficult breathing often. Smoking, other chest illnesses, exercise or anxiety can make a person with asthma wheeze. Sometimes patients who do not have asthma may wheeze. Pneumonia and bronchitis can also cause wheeze.

3. Bronchitis

Bronchitis is sometimes caused by a bacterial infection.
Almost all patients with bronchitis are aged 13 years or more.
A patient with bronchitis has a cough and coughs up sputum for 8 days or more. The sputum may be yellow, green or red. If the sputum is red, the patient may have tuberculosis.

4. Upper respiratory infection

Upper respiratory infections are very common. They are normally caused by viruses. Upper respiratory infections may cause a fever and cough. A patient may cough up sputum that is clear, white, green or yellow. Upper respiratory infections usually get better without medicines.

Tuberculosis is a separate type of chest problem and is covered in Lesson 12.

Chest illnesses in children aged 5 years or less

Make sure that each student has a copy of Appendix 1.

Taking a history and examining the patient

Ask the questions in Appendix 1. Make sure that the child does not have a general danger sign. Next, examine the child. Appendix 1 and the role play that we will now do tell you how to examine the patient and what to look for.

Ask three students to act out the demonstration as you read it to the class. Ask one student to play the role of the doctor, one to play the mother and a third student to play the child. Ask the students to sit at the front of the classroom. Tell the class who each student is pretending to be.

Demonstration

1. Make sure that the child is not crying or moving when you examine him. If the child is crying, ask the mother to breastfeed him or to hold him close. Do not touch the child.
2. Wait until the child is calm. Count how many times he breathes in one minute.
3. Ask the mother to lift the child's clothes from his chest. Look below the ribs to see if the skin is pulled in when the child breathes in. This is called chest indrawing.

Show the students a picture of a child with chest indrawing.

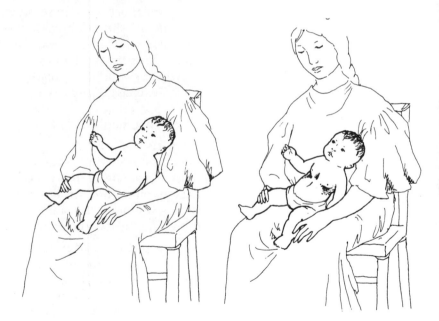

PICTURE 3 *Chest indrawing*

4. Listen for a noise when the child breathes *in*. If there is a hard noise, this is called stridor. If the child has stridor when he is calm, he may have epiglottitis (see Lesson 14). If he has stridor, give him an intramuscular injection of chloramphenicol (40 mg or 0.2 ml per kg body weight). Do not give more than 1000 mg (5.6 ml) of chloramphenicol. If there is no chloramphenicol, give benzylpenicillin. Next, send him to hospital immediately. **Do not put in a nasogastric tube**.

5. Listen for a noise when the child breathes out. If there is a soft whistling noise, or it is difficult for him to breathe out, he has wheeze.
6. Next, feel the child for fever and look for anaemia.

Thank the students who acted out the role play.

Diagnosis and treatment

Appendix 1 tells you how to diagnose and treat chest illnesses in children aged 5 years or less.

A severe illness which may be pneumonia or asthma

- If the child has chest indrawing or looks uncomfortable with fast breathing, he has a severe illness which may be pneumonia or asthma.
- If the child is aged less than 2 months and has stopped feeding well or breathes 60 times or more in one minute, he has a severe illness which may be pneumonia.

Give the child an injection of benzylpenicillin. Give 0.1 million IU (60 mg) for each kg of body weight. If the child has a fever, give the first-line malaria treatment in malaria areas. If the child has a wheeze, give a rapid acting bronchodilator. Next, send the child to hospital immediately.

Pneumonia which is not severe

- If a child has fast breathing he probably has pneumonia.
- If he does not have a general danger sign or a severe illness which may be pneumonia or asthma, the pneumonia is not yet severe.

POSTER 3:
(Prepared poster)

Fast breathing in children
Copy Table 1 onto Poster 3.

TABLE 1 Fast breathing in children

Age	Child has fast breathing if
Up to 2 months	60 breaths or more in one minute
2 months up to 12 months	50 breaths or more in one minute
12 months up to 5 years	40 breaths or more in one minute

If the child has fast breathing but looks comfortable, give co-trimoxazole or amoxicillin for 5 days. If the child has a fever in a malaria area, give co-trimoxazole. This is because co-trimoxazole can treat both pneumonia and malaria. (Chloroquine and Fansidar are better treatments for malaria.) Teach the mother about home care for a child with a chest illness (see below, p35). Ask her to bring the child back after 2 days.

If, after 2 days, the child has not improved or is worse, give an injection of benzylpenicillin and send him to hospital immediately.

No pneumonia

- **Upper respiratory infection**
  If the child does not have fast breathing, he does not have pneumonia. He probably has an upper respiratory infection. He may have a cough. Do not give an antibiotic. Teach the mother about home care of children with chest illnesses.

- **Wheeze**
  If this is the first time the child has had a wheeze, treat him for pneumonia. If the child has a wheeze and has had wheeze before, he probably has asthma. Treat the wheeze.

- **Ear or throat infection**
  If the child has an ear or throat problem, he may need an antibiotic (see Lesson 14).

- **Fever**
  If the child has a fever and there is malaria in your area, give the first-line malaria treatment.

Chest illness in an adult or a child aged 6 years or more

Make sure each student has a copy of Appendix 2.

Taking a history and examining the patient

Make sure that the patient does not have a general danger sign. Ask the questions in Appendix 2. Make sure that you also:
1. Ask the patient to cough. When the patient coughs, ask her to tell you if and where this causes pain.
2. Ask a patient who is aged 13 years or more: 'What colour is your sputum?'

Next, examine the patient. Appendix 2 tells you how to examine the patient and what to look for.

Ask two students to act out the following steps as you read them out. Ask one to play the doctor and one to play the patient. Ask the two students to sit at the front of the classroom. Tell the class who each student is pretending to be.

Demonstration

1. Feel for fever and look for anaemia.
2. Count how many times she breathes in one minute.
3. Look for chest indrawing.
4. Listen for stridor. If the patient has stridor (a hard noise when she breathes in), she may have epiglottitis. If she has stridor, give her an intramuscular injection of chloramphenicol (40 mg or 0.2 ml for each kg of body weight). Do not give more than

1000 mg (5.6 ml) of chloramphenicol. If there is no chloramphenicol, give benzylpenicillin. Next, send her to hospital immediately. **Do not put in a nasogastric tube**.

5. Listen for a wheeze. If the patient has wheeze and her record card tells you that she has asthma, give a rapid acting bronchodilator. Wait 15 minutes. Take a history and examine the patient. Then, treat the patient in the same way as any other patient with a chest illness.

6. If the patient has pain in the side of the chest (ribs) when she coughs, listen carefully to that part of the chest with a stethoscope. If you hear a crackle when she breathes in, she probably has pneumonia.

Diagnosis and treatment

Appendix 2 tells you how to diagnose and treat chest illnesses in patients aged 6 years or more.

A severe illness which may be pneumonia or asthma

- If the patient has a general danger sign, treat her for a very severe febrile disease.
- If the patient has stridor when calm, chest indrawing, looks uncomfortable with fast breathing or has blue lips, she has a severe illness which may be pneumonia.

Give the patient an injection of benzylpenicillin. Give 2 million IU (1200 mg). If the patient has a fever and there is malaria in your area, give a first-line malaria treatment. If the patient has wheeze, give a rapid acting bronchodilator. Next, send the patient to hospital immediately.

Pneumonia which is not severe

- If a patient has fast breathing and fever, she has pneumonia.
- If she has crackles in her lungs, she probably has pneumonia.

Give the patient amoxicillin or co-trimoxazole for 5 days. Tell the patient to come back to the health centre after 2 days, or before 2 days if she becomes more ill. If she is no better or gets worse, give her an injection of benzylpenicillin and send her to hospital immediately. If the patient's breathing is then slower but she has a fever, treat her for malaria in malaria areas. If the patient is taking co-trimoxazole, do not give her another malaria treatment.

POSTER 4:
(Prepared poster)

Fast breathing in patients over 6 years old
Copy Table 2 onto Poster 4.

TABLE 2 Fast breathing in patients over 6 years

Age	The patient has fast breathing if
6 years up to 12 years	30 breaths or more in one minute
13 years or more	25 breaths or more in one minute

No pneumonia

If the patient has no signs of very severe illness or pneumonia, she may have:

- **Wheeze**

  If this is the first time the patient has had a wheeze, treat her for pneumonia. If the patient has a wheeze and has had wheeze before, she probably has asthma. Treat the wheeze.

- **Bronchitis**

  If a patient aged 13 years or more has been coughing up yellow or green sputum for 8 days or more, treat her for bronchitis.

  If a patient has red sputum which is not caused by a nosebleed, treat her for bronchitis. Next, send her to the tuberculosis clinic or examine the sputum for acid fast bacilli (AFB). (Tuberculosis is covered in Lesson 12.)

  Treat the bronchitis with amoxicillin 250 mg three times a day for 5 days. If you do not have amoxicillin use co-trimoxazole. Use co-trimoxazole if the patient has a fever and might have malaria.

- **Upper respiratory infection**

  If the patient has a cough but no pneumonia, asthma or bronchitis, she probably has an upper respiratory infection. She may cough up coloured or clear sputum, but will not have fast breathing. Do not give an antibiotic. Teach the patient about home care for chest illnesses and advise her to eat a mixed diet.

  If the patient has an ear or throat problem, she may need an antibiotic.

- **Fever**

  If the patient has a fever and there is malaria in your area, give the first-line malaria treatment.

Give each student a copy of Tables 3, 4 and 5 and encourage questions.

TABLE 3 Antibiotics for pneumonia: amoxicillin

Age	Dose of amoxicillin
Up to 2 months	62.5 mg 3 times a day for 5 days (2.5 ml or ¼ tablet)
2 months up to 12 months	125 mg 3 times a day for 5 days (5 ml or ½ tablet)
12 months up to 10 years	250 mg 3 times a day for 5 days (10 ml or 1 tablet)
11 years and over	500 mg 3 times a day for 5 days (2 tablets)

TABLE 4   Antibiotics for pneumonia: co-trimoxazole

Age	Dose of co-trimoxazole
Up to 6 months	2.5 ml 2 times a day for 5 days (¼ tablet)
6 months up to 6 years	5 ml 2 times a day for 5 days (½ tablet)
6 years up to 13 years	1 tablet 2 times a day for 5 days
13 years and over	2 tablets 2 times a day for 5 days

TABLE 5   Antibiotics for pneumonia: benzylpenicillin

Age	Dose of benzylpenicillin
Up to 2 months	0.1 million IU for each kg of body weight then send to hospital
2 months up to 5 years	See above: amoxicillin or co-trimoxazole (Tables 3 and 4)
6 years up to 12 years	Only if severe pneumonia. 0.1 million IU for each kg of body weight but no more than 2 million IU
13 years and over	Only if severe pneumonia. 2 million IU

How to treat wheeze

If a patient has wheeze, you must decide first if she has respiratory distress. Patients with respiratory distress find it very difficult to breathe. Respiratory distress can be caused by pneumonia and asthma.

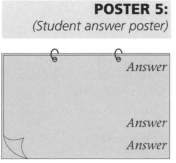

POSTER 5:
(Student answer poster)

Answer

Answer

Answer

Respiratory distress
Ask the students to tell you if they have seen patients with respiratory distress. Ask what they have seen.

The patient looks **uncomfortable** and has **fast breathing** (fast breathing in a patient who looks comfortable is *not* a sign of respiratory distress).

There is **chest indrawing**.

The patient is **not able to talk or feed**.

Treating wheeze when the patient has respiratory distress

- If a patient *with a wheeze* has any signs of respiratory distress, give her a rapid-acting bronchodilator, an injection of benzylpenicillin and send her to hospital immediately.

Commonly used rapid-acting bronchodilators are inhaled salbutamol or epinephrine injections. Give salbutamol from a metered-dose inhaler through a spacer. Shake the inhaler. Press the metered dose inhaler once for each time the patient breathes in five times. Repeat this ten times. Shake the inhaler each time. Give epinephrine by injection under the skin. The doses are given in Table 6.

Show your students how to make a spacer from a plastic bottle. Next, show them how to use it to give salbutamol (Picture 4). Give each student a copy of Appendix 3 'How to give injections'.

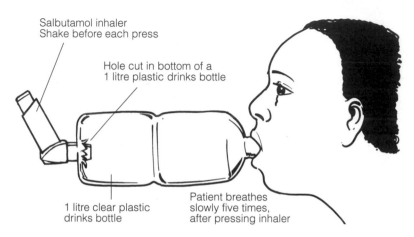

Salbutamol inhaler
Shake before each press

Hole cut in bottom of a
1 litre plastic drinks bottle

1 litre clear plastic
drinks bottle

Patient breathes
slowly five times,
after pressing inhaler

PICTURE 4 *How to use a salbutamol inhaler*

Treating wheeze when the patient has no respiratory distress

- If a patient with a wheeze has fast breathing, treat her for pneumonia which is not yet severe. These patients will not normally need a bronchodilator.
- If a patient who is not given antibiotics has a wheeze, give her a bronchodilator to use at home for 5 days. Teach the patient about home care for chest illnesses.
- Bronchodilators for use at home: aminophylline or oral salbutamol are slow-acting bronchodilators. The doses are given in Table 6. If possible, give treatment with a salbutamol metered-dose inhaler, used with a spacer, instead. Show the patient how to use the inhaler. Explain that she needs to press the metered dose inhaler two times every 4 hours.
- If this is the second time the patient has had a wheeze with no other signs of pneumonia, tell her that she has asthma. Do not forget that patients with asthma may become ill with severe asthma or pneumonia.

Give each student a copy of Table 6 and encourage them to ask questions.

TABLE 6 Bronchodilators

Age	Dose of aminophylline 100 mg tablet (slow-acting)
Up to 12 months	¼ tablet 3 times a day for 5 days
12 months up to 5 years	½ tablet 3 times a day for 5 days
6 years and over	1 tablet 3 times a day for 5 days
Age	**Dose of oral salbutamol 2 or 4 mg tablet (slow-acting)**
Up to 12 months	1 mg 3 times a day for 5 days
12 months up to 5 years	2 mg 3 times a day for 5 days
6 years and over	4 mg 3 times a day for 5 days
Age	**Dose of epinephrine (1:1000 = 0.1%) (subcutaneous) (rapid-acting)**
Up to 12 months	0.1 ml
12 months up to 5 years	0.25 ml (¼ vial)
6 years and over	0.5 ml (½ vial)

Home treatment for chest illnesses

POSTER 6:
(Student answer poster)

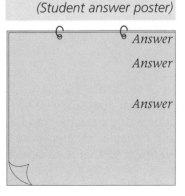

Answer

Answer

Answer

Home treatment for chest illnesses
Ask the students what patients can do at home for chest illnesses.

Give the patient **plenty of fluids.**

Continue to **feed** the patient **at least four times a day.** Feed children aged 5 or less **at least five times a day.**

Tell the patient to **come back** to the health centre **if** she has one of the following problems:
- **not able to drink**
- **breathing** becomes **difficult or fast**
- becomes **more ill**
- develops a **fever.**

SECTION 3: When to send patients to hospital

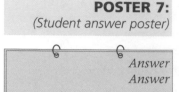

POSTER 7:
(Student answer poster)

When to send patients to hospital
Ask the students which patients must go to hospital.

Answer
Answer

Answer
Answer

1. patients with a **general danger sign**
2. patients with a **severe illness which may be pneumonia or asthma**
3. patients who have **stridor when calm**
4. patients with **respiratory distress**

Refreshment break

SECTION 4: Practical: examining real patients

In this section, the students practise their skills on the seven patients you have asked to come to the lesson.

■ You and the six students who have discussed each patient's symptoms, signs, diagnosis and treatment are the helpers.
■ Each helper and her patient will sit in a different part of the classroom.
■ Each helper will work with a small group of students to ask questions and examine one patient. The helper's job is to make sure that each group of students correctly finds the patient's symptoms and signs and decides on a diagnosis and treatment.
■ Divide the class into seven groups. Give the groups 20 minutes to see each patient. After they have examined one patient, ask the groups of students to move on to the next patient. All the groups should examine all seven patients.
■ Tell the students to use Appendix 1 and Appendix 2 to help them to ask questions, look for general danger signs, examine and decide how to treat each patient.

SECTION 5: Answers to the quiz

Ask the students to call out the answers to each question in the quiz. If the answers show that some students do not understand a point, ask a student who does understand to explain the point to the other students. Summarise the answer next to the questions on Poster 1.

1. If a patient is ill, he may breathe fast. How many breaths in one minute is fast breathing:

   For a child up to 2 months?
   60 breaths or more in one minute

For a child aged 2 months up to 12 months?
50 breaths or more in one minute

For a child aged 12 months up to 5 years?
40 breaths or more in one minute

For a child aged 6 years up to 12 years?
30 breaths or more in one minute

For an adult?
25 breaths or more in one minute

2. What would make you think that a patient had a severe illness which may be pneumonia or asthma?
The patient has: chest indrawing, stridor when calm, respiratory distress.
The patient is a child less than 2 months old who is breathing 60 times or more in one minute.

3. Patients who find it very difficult to breathe have respiratory distress. What are the signs of respiratory distress?
The patient looks uncomfortable and has fast breathing, or
There is chest indrawing, or
The patient is not able to talk or feed

4. A patient has a cough. She feeds well. She does not have chest indrawing. She does not have fast breathing. There is no noise when she breathes in or out. She has a fever. When she coughs there is no pain in the side of chest. She is not anaemic.
What illness(es) does she have?
Upper respiratory infection. She may also have malaria, if there is malaria in the area.
What treatment should you give her?
The patient does not need an antibiotic, unless she has an ear or throat problem. Treat for malaria if there is malaria in the area. Teach the patient or the mother about home treatment for chest illnesses.

Lesson 3 — Fever, malaria, convulsions and meningitis

BEFORE THE LESSON

- There are eight posters in this lesson. (See p. 4 for information on how to use the posters.)
  Prepared posters: 1, 4, 8
  Student answer posters: 2, 5, 6, 7
  Summary poster: 3

- Give one student a copy of the demonstration in this lesson. Practise the demonstration before the lesson. You need a pen, a patient record card and a child growth chart.

- Give each student a copy of Tables 1 and 2, summarising the doses of chloroquine or Fansidar.

- Prepare one copy of the discussion about patients in section 5 for each group of five students. For example, if you have 25 students, you will need five copies.

- Ask the students to bring their copy of Chapter 2 to the lesson.

- Cross out the box of advice about the first-line malaria treatment that does *not* apply in your country.

SECTION 1:   Quiz

POSTER 1:
(Prepared poster)

Quiz
Cross out the first-line malaria treatment that is *not* used in your country. Ask the students to answer the questions on their own. Do not give the answers until the end of the lesson.

> 1. What are the four general danger signs?
>
> 2. If the patient has a general danger sign, Kernig's sign or a fever with a stiff neck, what six things will you do?
>
> 3. What is chloroquine-resistant malaria? What is Fansidar-resistant malaria?
>
> 4. The following patients all have meningitis. What could you find when you take a history or examine them?
>   - a child aged 2 months
>   - a child aged 3 years
>   - a woman aged 31 years

SECTION 2:   Diagnosis and management of malaria

Section 2 starts with a demonstration. Ask a student to play a woman with a baby. You will play the doctor. Make sure you have a pen, a patient record card and a child growth chart. Say the lines slowly and loudly so that the class can hear.

The doctor sits near to a mother with her child in a health centre.

Demonstration

Doctor: Good morning.
Mother: Good morning.
Doctor: Please take a seat.
Mother: Thank you.
Doctor: Who is ill today?
Mother: My child Pili Tatu.
Doctor: How old is she?
Mother: One year old.
Doctor: What is wrong with her?
Mother: She has had a fever for two days.
Doctor: Anything else?
Mother: She is not feeding well and she vomited once this morning.
Doctor: Has she had a convulsion?
Mother: No, she's just not herself.
Doctor: Does she have a cough?
Mother: No.
Doctor: Does she have diarrhoea?
Mother: No.

The doctor examines the child.

Doctor: She has a high fever. Your child has malaria. May I see her growth chart? I see she has had all her vaccinations. She weighs 9 kg.

Cross out the box below that does not apply in your country.

> **If the first-line malaria treatment in your country is chloroquine:**
>
> Doctor: Your child needs to take chloroquine. Give her two teaspoonfuls now, two tomorrow, and one the day after tomorrow.
> *Mother: Yes I will.*
> Doctor: Can you tell me what I have asked you to do?
> *Mother: Give two teaspoonfuls today, two tomorrow and two the day after tomorrow.*
> Doctor: No. Two today, two tomorrow and one the day after tomorrow.
> *Mother: Oh. Two today, two tomorrow and one the day after tomorrow.*
> Doctor: That is correct.

If the first-line malaria treatment in your country is Fansidar:

Doctor: Your child has malaria. I am going to give her $\frac{1}{2}$ tablet of Fansidar before she leaves the health centre.

Mother: *Thank you.*

Doctor: Now I will show you how to bring her temperature down. It is important that the child does not get very hot. If the child gets hot, take her clothes off. Put a cloth in warm water. Wipe her body to keep the skin wet until the fever has gone. This will take less than 30 minutes. If the child vomits within one hour of taking the medicine, bring her back to the health centre. If she is still hot after two days, bring her back to the health centre.

Mother: *Thank you.*

Doctor: Now we will give her the first dose of her malaria medicine before you leave the health centre.

Ask your students: What did you think about that consultation? Look for the following answer:

Answer The communication was very good.

Ask your students: Why do you think the communication was good? Look for the following answers:

Answer The doctor and the child's mother sat close to each other.
Answer The doctor greeted the mother.
Answer The doctor was interested in the patient's problem.
Answer The doctor explained the medicine and the treatment.

Ask your students: What will be the result of this good communication? Look for the following answers:

Answer The mother will understand how to give the medicine.
Answer If the child does not get better after 2 days, the mother will bring the child back to see the doctor.
Answer The mother knows how to do tepid sponging.
Answer The mother is now less worried.

Fever

Fever is usually caused by the patient's body fighting against an infection.
- If fever is caused by a serious infection, for example malaria or pneumonia, the infections must be treated.
- If fever is caused by an infection that is not serious, for example an upper respiratory infection, the infection does not need treatment.

In many areas of the world, malaria is the most common serious cause of fever. Malaria is caused by malaria parasites. The parasites get into the body if a person is bitten by a mosquito that has malaria parasites.

*If you live in an area where there is no malaria, **do not** treat patients with a malaria treatment. If the patient has been in an area where there is malaria, then follow the advice given below.*

Treatment of fever

The most important thing to do is to treat the cause of the fever. Check first to see if a patient has a general danger sign, Kernig's sign or a stiff neck. These signs mean that the patient may have severe malaria, pneumonia or meningitis. These serious infections may be causing his fever. If there is a general danger sign, Kernig's sign or a stiff neck, treat the patient for a very severe febrile disease.

POSTER 2:
(Student answer poster)

The four general danger signs
Ask your students: What are the four general danger signs?
(The correct answers are in Chapter 2, see p. 7.)

POSTER 3:
(Summary poster)

Fever

1. Take a history and examine the patient. If you think that the patient has pneumonia, **treat** the **pneumonia immediately** in the health centre.

2. (a) In areas where there is *no malaria:*
   - If the patient does not have a general danger sign, **treat** the **cause of** the **fever**. Bring down a **high fever** (38.5°C or more under the arm) by **tepid sponging** and give a single dose of **paracetamol** in the health centre. Tell the patient to go to hospital if the fever is no better after 5 days.
   - If the patient has recently been in an area where there is malaria, treat for malaria immediately.

   (b) In areas where there is *malaria:*
   - **Treat for malaria** (or examine the blood for malaria parasites immediately) if a patient is a **child under 5 years old** or a **pregnant woman** and has had a **fever** in the **last 3 days**.
   - **Treat** all other patients **for malaria** only **if** you can find **no other cause for** the **fever**.
   - Bring down a high fever by **tepid sponging** and give a single dose of **paracetamol at** the **health centre**. After the fever has come down, give the first-line malaria treatment (either **chloroquine** or **Fansidar** tablets).

(*continued*)

- If you think a child or a pregnant woman has pneumonia and malaria, treat with co-trimoxazole instead of chloroquine or Fansidar. Co-trimoxazole can treat both pneumonia and malaria.
- If you have done a blood test to confirm a malaria diagnosis, and the patient also has pneumonia, give the first-line malaria treatment and an antibiotic for the pneumonia.

3. **Teach** mothers to treat a fever by **tepid sponging**.

4. **If** the patient **vomits less than one hour after** taking the **tablets**, bring down the fever by **tepid sponging**. Next, give him the **same dose again**.

5. Look for the measles rash. A patient who has fever and a rash all over his body may have measles. The rash does *not* itch. Diagnose measles if the patient also has red eyes *or* a cough *or* fluid coming from the nose.
   - If a patient has **measles, give** him **vitamin A**.
   - If a patient has had measles in the last 3 months, give him vitamin A.

If a patient has measles, look at the corneas in the eyes. If a **cornea is not clear**, treat the eyes with **tetracycline eye ointment**, give an intramuscular injection of benzylpenicillin, and send the patient to **hospital**.

First-line malaria treatment

The first-line treatment for malaria is either chloroquine or Fansidar (pyrimethamine and sulfadoxine). The national drug policy in each country will prescribe what the first-line malaria treatment is. Chloroquine is given in three doses on 3 days. Fansidar is given as one dose.

Cross out the box below that does not apply in your country.

POSTER 4:
(Prepared poster)

Dose of chloroquine

- On the **first day** give **10 mg for each kg** of body weight.
- On the **second day** give **10 mg for each kg** of body weight.
- On the **third day** give **5 mg for each kg** of body weight.
- Do not give more than 600 mg on the first and second days. Do not give more than 300 mg on the third day.
- Always tell the patient that chloroquine may make his skin itch.

If chloroquine is the first-line malaria treatment used in your country, give each student a copy of Table 1. Encourage them to ask questions about the table.

If your students need a way to measure liquid medicines, teach Appendix 5.

TABLE 1 Dose of chloroquine

Weight	Liquid			Give patient Total (in ml)	Tablets		
	Day				**Day**		
	1	**2**	**3**		**1**	**2**	**3**
2.5 kg or less	$\frac{1}{2}$ teaspoon	$\frac{1}{2}$ teaspoon	$\frac{1}{4}$ teaspoon	6.25 ml	$\frac{1}{4}$ tablet	$\frac{1}{4}$ tablet	$\frac{1}{4}$ tablet
2.6–5 kg	1 teaspoon	1 teaspoon	$\frac{1}{2}$ teaspoon	12.5 ml	$\frac{1}{2}$ tablet	$\frac{1}{2}$ tablet	$\frac{1}{4}$ tablet
5.1–7.5 kg	$1\frac{1}{2}$ teaspoons	$1\frac{1}{2}$ teaspoons	1 teaspoon	20 ml	$\frac{1}{2}$ tablet	$\frac{1}{2}$ tablet	$\frac{1}{4}$ tablet
7.6–10 kg	2 teaspoons	2 teaspoons	1 teaspoon	25 ml	1 tablet	1 tablet	$\frac{1}{2}$ tablet
10.1–12.5 kg	$2\frac{1}{2}$ teaspoons	$2\frac{1}{2}$ teaspoons	$1\frac{1}{2}$ teaspoons	32.5 ml	1 tablet	1 tablet	$\frac{1}{2}$ tablet
12.6–15 kg					1 tablet	1 tablet	$\frac{1}{2}$ tablet
15.5–22.5 kg					$1\frac{1}{2}$ tablets	$1\frac{1}{2}$ tablets	1 tablet
23–30 kg					2 tablets	2 tablets	1 tablet
30.5–37.5 kg					$2\frac{1}{2}$ tablets	$2\frac{1}{2}$ tablets	$1\frac{1}{2}$ tablets
38–45 kg					3 tablets	3 tablets	$1\frac{1}{2}$ tablets
45.5 kg or more					4 tablets	4 tablets	2 tablets

Notes about the table:
- Each 5 ml teaspoon of liquid is assumed to contain 50 mg chloroquine base.
- Each tablet is assumed to contain 150 mg of chloroquine base.

Remember that:
- 1 teaspoon holds about 5 ml of liquid medicine.
- $\frac{1}{2}$ teaspoon holds 2.5 ml of liquid medicine.
- $\frac{1}{4}$ teaspoon holds 1.25 ml of liquid medicine.

If Fansidar is the first-line malaria treatment used in your country, give each student a copy of Table 2. Encourage them to ask questions about the table.

TABLE 2 Doses of Fansidar

Fansidar is given in one dose, immediately. The dose of Fansidar depends on the age of the patient.	
Age	**Dose of Fansidar (pyrimethamine with sulfadoxine)**
Up to 4 years old	$\frac{1}{2}$ tablet
4–6 years old	1 tablet
7–9 years old	$1\frac{1}{2}$ tablets
10–14 years old	2 tablets
15 years old and over	3 tablets

Malaria which is resistant to the first-line malaria treatment

Some malaria parasites are resistant to the first-line malaria treatment. If parasites are resistant, this means the treatment will not kill all of them.

The next two boxes tell you about chloroquine-resistant malaria and Fansidar-resistant malaria. The boxes tell you how to diagnose malaria that is resistant to first-line medicines and what treatment to give patients with resistant malaria.

Cross out the box that does not apply in your country.

Chloroquine-resistant malaria

Ask your students what chloroquine-resistant malaria is. Look for the following answer:

Answer Some malaria parasites have learned how to defend themselves against chloroquine. This means that chloroquine does not kill all the malaria parasites. To kill these resistant malaria parasites, you must use another malaria treatment.

Ask your students if this means that every time that this patient gets malaria they need to be treated with Fansidar or quinine. Look for the following answer:

Answer No. Each mosquito bite can give a person either normal malaria or chloroquine-resistant malaria parasites. If a patient does not have a fever for 2 weeks or more, the chloroquine-resistant malaria parasites are all dead. If the patient gets malaria again, it is because more malaria parasites have entered the body from a new mosquito bite. Treat the patient with chloroquine first.

(*continued*)

Ask your students how they can tell if a patient has chloroquine-resistant malaria. Look for the following answer:

Answer A patient has chloroquine-resistant malaria if they have a fever caused by malaria for more than 2 days *and* less than 14 days after starting chloroquine.

Ask your students what they should do if a patient with fever is treated with chloroquine but does not get better. Look for the following answers:

Answer First, look again for another cause of the fever. Take the patient's history. Examine the patient.

Answer If you can find no other cause for the fever, treat the patient with a second-line malaria treatment.

Answer If possible, send the patient to a hospital where the patient can have a blood test to look for malaria parasites. If this blood test shows that the patient has malaria, they have chloroquine-resistant malaria. Give him a second-line malaria treatment, for example Fansidar or quinine.

Answer If a patient still has a fever 2 days after treatment with a second-line malaria treatment, send them to hospital. The patient may have typhoid fever, relapsing fever, kala azar or another infection which is causing the fever.

Fansidar-resistant malaria

Ask the students what Fansidar-resistant malaria is. Look for the following answer:

Answer Some malaria parasites have learned how to defend themselves against Fansidar. This means that Fansidar does not kill all of the malaria parasites. To kill these malaria parasites, you need to use another malaria treatment.

Ask the students if this means that every time that this patient gets malaria, he needs to be treated with quinine. Look for the following answer:

Answer No. Each mosquito bite can carry either normal or Fansidar-resistant malaria parasites. If a patient does not have a fever for 2 weeks or more, the Fansidar-resistant malaria parasites are all dead. If the patient gets malaria again, it is usually the result of more malaria parasites entering the body from a new mosquito bite. Treat the patient with Fansidar first.

Ask the students how they can tell if a patient has Fansidar-resistant malaria.

(continued)

Answer A patient has Fansidar-resistant malaria if he has a fever caused by malaria for more than 2 days *and* less than 14 days after starting Fansidar.

Ask your students what they should do if a patient with fever is treated with Fansidar but does not get better. Look for the following answers:

Answer First, look again for another cause for the patient's fever. Take the patient's history. Examine the patient.

Answer If you can find no other cause for his fever, treat the patient with second-line malaria treatment.

Answer If possible, send the patient to a hospital where he can have a blood test to look for malaria parasites. If this blood test shows that the patient has malaria, he has Fansidar-resistant malaria. Give him a second-line malaria treatment, for example quinine.

Answer If a patient still has a fever 2 days after treatment with a second-line malaria treatment, send him to hospital. He may have typhoid fever, relapsing fever, kala azar or another infection which is causing the fever.

SECTION 3: Diagnosis and management of convulsions, meningitis and cerebral malaria

Convulsions

Cerebral malaria, meningitis or a high fever can cause convulsions. A patient having a convulsion becomes stiff and may shake. She is not able to stop the stiffness or shaking.

POSTER 5:
(Student answer poster)

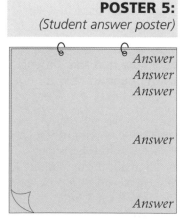

Causes of convulsions
Ask the students: What causes convulsions?

Answer **Cerebral malaria**.

Answer **Meningitis**.

Answer **A high fever**. Many illnesses cause a high fever. A child may have a febrile convulsion if her fever becomes high very quickly. Only children less than 5 years old have febrile convulsions.

Answer **Low blood sugar**. This is called hypoglycaemia. Patients with very severe febrile disease get hypoglycaemia. A patient with diabetes may also get hypoglycaemia if she takes too much insulin or too many diabetes tablets.

Answer **Epilepsy**. (See Lesson 11.)

Ask your students: How can we prevent a patient with a fever or a general danger sign from having a convulsion? Look for the following answers:

Answer   **Tepid sponging** can prevent some convulsions caused by fever, because tepid sponging cools the body.

Answer   A single dose of **paracetamol** in the health centre helps to cool the body.

Answer   **Treat** a patient with a general danger sign **to prevent low blood sugar**.

Ask your students how they would treat a patient who has had a convulsion in the past 24 hours. Look for the following answer:

Answer   The convulsion may be caused by severe malaria or meningitis. Treat in the same way as you would treat a patient who has a very severe febrile disease (see Chapter 2). This treatment may cure severe malaria, pneumonia or meningitis.

Cerebral malaria

Cerebral malaria is a serious illness that damages the brain. It is caused by a type of malaria called *falciparum malaria*. Giving the correct treatment as soon as possible will save many lives. Children less than 5 years old and women who are pregnant for the first time get cerebral malaria more than other patients. The symptoms of cerebral malaria may be the same as symptoms of meningitis. You do not need to know whether a patient has cerebral malaria or meningitis to decide about treatment.

Ask your students how they would treat a patient with symptoms of cerebral malaria or meningitis. Look for the following answer:

Answer   Both illnesses are treated in the same way as a very severe febrile disease.

Meningitis

Meningitis is a serious illness that damages the brain. It can be caused by infection with bacteria or a virus. Giving the correct treatment as soon as possible will save many lives. However, some patients will die from meningitis, even if they get the correct treatment.

POSTER 6:
(Student answer poster)

Signs of meningitis in patients aged under 6 months
A patient aged under 6 months has meningitis. Ask your students: What might you find when you take a history or examine him?

Answer   **Convulsions**.
Answer   **Fever**.
Answer   The child is **unable to breastfeed**.
Answer   **Vomiting**.

POSTER 7:
(Student answer poster)

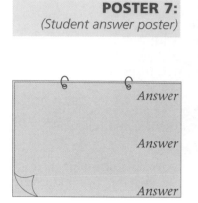

Answer

Answer

Answer

Answer

Signs of meningitis in patients aged more than 6 months

A patient aged more than 6 months has meningitis. Ask your students: What might you find when you take a history or examine her?

A **stiff neck**. If a child can move and bend her neck, she does not have a stiff neck. Tickle the patient's toes to encourage her to look down.

Look for **Kernig's sign**. Kernig's sign is a pain felt in the back, neck or head when the patient's hip is bent and the knee straightened.

Convulsions, fever or **vomiting**.

Ask the students how they would treat a patient with symptoms of meningitis. Look for the following answer:

Treat all patients who have a general danger sign, a stiff neck, or Kernig's sign with the treatment for a very severe febrile disease.

Show the students how to look for Kernig's sign. Ask your students to tell you what six things they should do if a patient has a very severe febrile disease, or a stiff neck or Kernig's sign. The answers are in Chapter 2.

Refreshment break

SECTION 4: When to send patients to hospital

POSTER 8:
(Prepared poster)

When to send patients to hospital

> **Send** patients with a fever **to hospital**:
> 1. if the patient has one of the four **general danger signs**, **Kernig's sign** or a **stiff neck**
> 2. if the patient has **severe anaemia**
> 3. if the patient has **jaundice**
> 4. if the fever is **no better 2 days after treatment** with the first-line malaria treatment – for a malaria blood test
> 5. if a patient still has a **fever 2 days after treatment with a second malaria treatment**.

SECTION 5: Practical – discussion about patients

Divide the students into groups of five or six. Give each group of students a copy of the following questions. Tell the students that this activity will show them how to treat three patients with common illnesses. The students have 30 minutes to decide what illness each patient has and what treatment to give each patient. (If there is no malaria in your country give patients 1 and 2 in the following examples other illnesses that cause a fever.)

Activity

Patient 1

A 2-year-old girl has had a fever and diarrhoea for the last 2 days. Today she has had diarrhoea three times, but she does not have a fever. The girl is not anaemic and not dehydrated. She weighs 13 kg.
1. What illness does the girl have?
2. How will you treat her?
3. What advice will you give her mother?

Patient 2

A 5-year-old boy was treated with the first-line malaria treatment 9 days ago. The boy has a fever and a cough. He is able to drink. He breathes 30 times in one minute. He does not have chest indrawing. There is no noise when he breathes in or out. He is not anaemic. He weighs 17 kg.
1. What illness does the boy have?
2. How will you treat him?
3. What advice will you give his mother?

Patient 3

A 4-month-old boy has had a fever for one day. He has had a convulsion. He has vomited once. He is not breastfeeding well. He has a high fever. He moves less than usual when awake but he is not having a convulsion now.
1. What illness does he have?
2. How will you treat him?

Answers

Ask the students to call out their answers. Give them the correct answers:

Patient 1

1. What illness does the girl have?
   Malaria.

2. How will you treat her?
   Chloroquine 150 mg/150 mg/75 mg or Fansidar $\frac{1}{2}$ tablet.

3. What advice will you give her mother?
   Advise her to do tepid sponging to reduce the fever. If the patient vomits within one hour of taking the medicine, the mother should bring her back to the health centre. If she is still hot after 2 days, return to the health centre.

Patient 2

1. What illness does the boy have?
   The boy may have malaria which is resistant to the first-line malaria treatment.

2. How will you treat him?
   Send him to hospital for a malaria blood test.

3. What advice will you give his mother?
   Advise her to do tepid sponging. She should give the

child a mixed diet five times a day or more until he is well again and continue to feed the child five times a day for a week after he gets well.

Patient 3

1. What illness does he have?
   A very severe febrile disease.

2. What should his treatment be?
   If he has vomited, clear his mouth with your finger. Lay him on his side.
   Use tepid sponging to reduce the fever.
   Treat the patient to prevent low blood sugar: give 30–50 ml of expressed breastmilk or milk or sugar-water, using a cup and spoon.

   > *If there is malaria in the area, give him an intramuscular injection of quinine or chloroquine.*

   Give the patient an intramuscular injection of chloramphenicol, benzylpenicillin or procaine penicillin fortified.
   Send him to hospital immediately.

SECTION 6: Answers to the quiz

Ask the students to call out the answers to each question in the quiz.

1. What are the four general danger signs?
   See answers in Chapter 2, see p. 7.

2. If patient has a general danger sign, a stiff neck or Kernig's sign what six things will you do?
   See answers in Chapter 2, see p. 8.

3. What is chloroquine-resistant malaria? What is Fansidar-resistant malaria?
   Some malaria parasites have learned how to defend themselves against malaria treatment such as chloroquine or Fansidar. This means that not all of the malaria parasites are killed by the medicine. To kill these malaria parasites it is necessary to use another malaria treatment such as quinine.

4. The following patients all have meningitis. What might you find when you take a history or examine the patient?

   2-month-old child: **a general danger sign, fever**
   3-year-old child: **a stiff neck, Kernig's sign, a general danger sign, fever**
   31-year-old woman: **a stiff neck, Kernig's sign, a general danger sign, fever**

Lesson 4 — Malnutrition and anaemia

BEFORE THE LESSON

- This is a long lesson. Make sure that the students can stay for 6–7 hours. Plan to have at least one refreshment break during the lesson in addition to a lunch break.

- There are 13 posters in this lesson. (See p. 4 for information on how to use the posters.)
  Prepared posters: 1, 3, 6, 7, 10, 12, 13.
  Student answer posters: 2, 4, 5, 8, 9, 11.

- Prepare a copy of Appendix 6 for each student.

- Prepare five copies of Appendix 7.

- Prepare the role plays. Write the information for the patient, the doctor and the observer on separate pieces of paper. Use a paper clip to keep each role play together. You need six copies of each role play, one copy for each of six groups of students. Prepare six copies of the growth charts in Pictures 11, 12 and 13 using real growth charts.

- If the direct recording scale is used in your country, you will need a direct recording scale, a pen, a bucket of water, two cups and some string.

- If you *do not* use direct recording scale, fill in the last two weights in the growth chart for role play 4 (Picture 13). Juanita Garcia Lopez's growth line has gone down on the two most recent weighings.

- Cut out 10 triangles and 7 circles from paper for the activity in section 3.

- In Table 3 cross out the box of advice about the first-line malaria treatment that does not apply in your country.

- If tablets that combine ferrous sulphate 200 mg (60 mg iron) and folic acid 0.25 mg are available, recommend this combination to treat anaemia instead of ferrous sulphate 200 mg.

SECTION 1: Quiz

POSTER 1:
(Prepared poster)

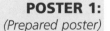

Quiz

Copy the *growth lines only* from the growth charts in Pictures 5, 6, 7 (see page 56) into the poster below question 1. Ask the students to answer the questions on their own. Do not give the answers until the end of the lesson.

1. What do the following growth lines mean? What will you do for each child?
2. What are the six rules of good nutrition?
3. What happens to a child who is not given food which follows the six rules of good nutrition?
4. What are the causes of anaemia?

SECTION 2:   Diagnosis and management of malnutrition

People need to eat a mixed diet that includes different types of food. A mixed diet helps people to work, grow and fight illness. People get malnutrition if they do not eat enough of the right foods.

Eating a mixed diet is very important for children aged less than 5 years. Children with malnutrition do not grow and are more likely to get ill. A mixed diet is also important for young women and women who are pregnant or breastfeeding. A mixed diet helps them to stay well and to have healthy babies. As well as a good diet, it is also good to advise women to wait for 2 or 3 years between pregnancies. During this time, a mixed diet will help their bodies become strong again to have a healthy baby and to produce nutritious breast milk.

Eating a mixed diet

People need food that gives them energy, protein, vitamins, minerals and carbohydrate.

Energy

Children need food containing energy when they are growing.

You can make sure children get enough energy by:
- giving them four or more meals of carbohydrate food every day
- adding foods that contain large amounts of energy to some or all of a child's meals.

Protein

Children must eat protein at least one time every day to help them to grow.

Vitamins and minerals

Vitamins and minerals help children to grow and help adults and children to fight infections. Iron is a mineral we need in order to make haemoglobin. Vitamin C and folic acid are important vitamins. Vitamin C helps our bodies to use the iron in food. Unfortunately, drinking tea or coffee with meals prevents our bodies from using iron.

POSTER 2:
(Student answer poster)

Examples of nutritious foods
Ask the students what local foods contain large amounts of energy, protein, vitamins, minerals and carbohydrate.
Table 1 below gives examples of correct answers. Choose the foods from Table 1 which are available in your area.

TABLE 1   Examples of nutritious foods

Nutritional benefit	Examples of foods
Energy	Cooking oil, sugar, palm oil, groundnut oil and fried foods
Protein	Breastmilk, beans, lentils and fish. Liver, kidney, blood, eggs, grasshoppers, locusts, crickets and termites
Vitamin C	Fresh fruit, lightly-cooked vegetables and dark green leafy vegetables
Folic acid	Breastmilk, beans, groundnuts, lentils, dark green leafy vegetables, liver and kidney
Iron	Small whole fish, fish and dark green leafy vegetables. Liver, kidney, blood, eggs, grasshoppers locusts, crickets and termites
Carbohydrate	Maize, cassava, rice and potatoes

POSTER 3:
(Prepared poster)

How to prevent malnutrition

Advise:

- **Children** and **pregnant women** to **eat four meals a day**
- **Everyone** to **eat protein** foods at least **one time every day**
- **Everyone** to **eat** dark green leafy **vegetables, fruit** or lightly cooked vegetables at least **two times a day**

Six rules of good nutrition

People have malnutrition because they are poor or because they do not know how to eat a mixed diet. Health workers cannot prevent poverty, but they can tell people how to eat a mixed diet to prevent malnutrition.

If you are a health worker you can:
- Teach by example, by giving your own family a mixed diet.
- Arrange cooking demonstrations to show people how to make nutritious meals.
- Advise people about good local foods that are not expensive.
- Help people to grow local crops that are part of a mixed diet.
- Teach people about the six rules of good nutrition.

POSTER 4:
(Student answer poster)

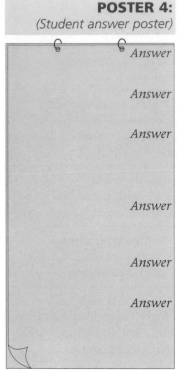

Answer

Answer

Answer

Answer

Answer

Answer

The six rules of good nutrition
Ask the students: What are the six rules of good nutrition?

1. Continue to **breastfeed** children **until** they are **2 years** old. Breastfeed **at least six times a day**.

2. Give some **soft foods,** (for example maize or cassava porridge) **in addition to breastmilk after** the child is **5 months old.**

3. Give **protein foods** (for example beans, little fish or groundnuts) **in addition to breastmilk after** the child is **6 months old.** Mash or crush these foods until the child is 12 months old, to help him to eat them.

4. Give **vegetables and fruit in addition to breastmilk after** the child is **6 months old.** Mash or crush these foods until the child is 12 months old.

5. Give **all children over** the age of **9 months** at least **four meals a day in addition to breastmilk.**

6. **Give ill children more food** than usual. Feed ill children who are more than 9 months old five times a day. Breastfeed all ill children who are less than 2 years old at least eight times a day. Continue to feed the child more often until the child is well again and for one extra week.

Mothers will learn more if you help them to prepare foods which follow the six rules of good nutrition. Ask mothers to repeat the rules of good nutrition to you.

When do children get malnutrition?

Children are more likely to get malnutrition at particular times. We have called these danger times. If we know when children are in danger of getting malnutrition, we can teach mothers how to prevent it.

POSTER 5:
(Student answer poster)

Malnutrition danger times for children
Ask the students when children are in danger of getting malnutrition.
Table 2 lists the danger times.

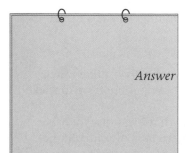

Answer

TABLE 2   Malnutrition danger times for children

Danger time	Reason
Before birth	If a **pregnant woman** has a **poor diet**, the baby does not grow well inside the woman. The woman is also not able to make enough breastmilk to feed her new baby.

TABLE 2 *(continued)*

	Danger time	Reason
Answer	**8 to 10 months**	If a child is **only** fed with **breastmilk**, he will not grow **as well as** he should. He needs other foods in addition to breast milk from 5 months of age.
Answer	If the mother gets **pregnant again**	She **may stop breastfeeding**. Breastfeeding when pregnant does *not* harm the child or the unborn baby.
Answer	**After the mother stops breast-feeding**	Breastmilk contains protein, energy, vitamins and minerals. If a child does not eat a mixed diet he **will not get** enough **protein, energy, vitamins** and **minerals**.
Answer	The baby is **bottle-fed**	Breastmilk is free, clean and protects children from diarrhoea. Milk from a **bottle** often has **bacteria** in it which cause **diarrhoea** and weight loss.
Answer	**Another baby** is born	The mother has less time for the older child and **stops breastfeeding** him.
Answer	The family is not able to get **food** because of famine, war or poverty	The child receives **less food**. The food that the child receives is **not** a **mixed diet**.

Early malnutrition

Diagnosing and treating early malnutrition can save a child's life. It prevents the child from getting more severe malnutrition. Early malnutrition is easier to treat than severe malnutrition.

Growth charts

Growth charts show the mother and the health worker how well children are growing. A child's growth chart tells you if a child has early malnutrition.

If direct recording scales are used in your country, show the students what they looks like. Explain how the direct recording scales work.

<table>
<tr><td>

POSTER 6:
(Prepared poster)

</td><td>

Growth lines
Copy Pictures 5, 6 and 7 onto poster 6.

</td></tr>
</table>

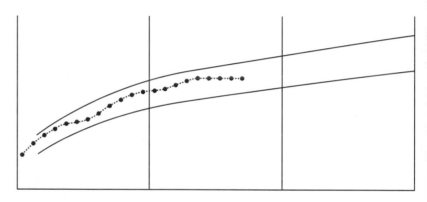

PICTURE 5   *Growth chart of a child who is growing*

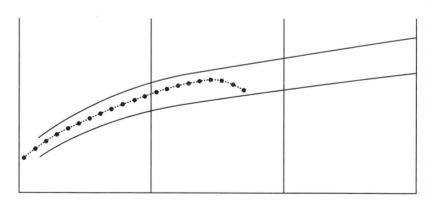

PICTURE 6   *Growth chart of a child who is not growing*

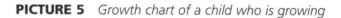

PICTURE 7   *Growth chart of a child who is losing weight*

Explain to the students that the line on a growth chart tells the health worker and the mother how well the child is growing. Tell the students that it is the *direction* of the line that is important.

• If the line is going up: the child is gaining weight and growing.

- If the line is flat: the child is not gaining weight and is not growing.
- If the line is going down: the child is losing weight and is not growing.

Diagnosing malnutrition early

POSTER 7: _(Prepared poster)_

Diagnosing malnutrition early

1. Weigh all children under 5 years of age at the Maternal and Child Health clinic. **Weigh children under** the age of **2** years **every month. Weigh children over** the age of **2** years **every 3 months**.

2. Each time you see a child under the age of **5** years at your health centre, **look at** the child's **growth chart**.

3. If the **growth line** is **flat or going down**, treat the child for early malnutrition.

4. If the **growth line has gone down at the two most recent weighings**, or the child has swelling of the legs, he may have severe malnutrition. Send him to the nutrition clinic.

Treating early malnutrition

- **Take the patient's history**.
- Ask the mother if she has stopped breastfeeding or if the child is not eating a mixed diet.
- **Treat** any **illness** that you find.
- **Teach** the child's mother the **six rules of good nutrition**.
- If the child is 1 year old or more, give him 100 mg **mebendazole** two times a day for 3 days. Mebendazole is a treatment for worms. Do not give mebendazole if the child has been given mebendazole in the last 6 months.

Severe malnutrition

Diagnosing severe malnutrition

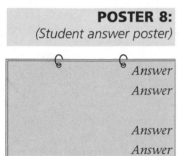

POSTER 8: _(Student answer poster)_

Signs of malnutrition in children

Ask the students What do children with severe malnutrition look like?

Answer   They have wasted and **thin muscles.**

Answer   They have little fat underneath the skin and it is easy to see the **bones**.

Answer   They have **thin**, straight, and sometimes red **hair**.

Answer   They have mouth and skin **ulcers.**

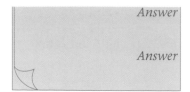

Answer

Answer

They look sad, **do not smile**, and have **no interest** in what is going on around them.

They may have **swelling** of the **legs** and **under** their **eyes**. This is called **kwashiorkor**. The swelling is caused by fluid under the skin which hides the thin muscles and bones.

Kwashiorkor

To tell if child has kwashiorkor, press the front of the lower part of the child's leg with your finger for 10 seconds. If, after you remove your finger, you can see where you were pressing, the child has fluid under his skin. Send all patients with fluid under the skin to **hospital immediately**. Without treatment most children with kwashiorkor will die.

Show Pictures 8 and 9 to the students. The child on the left has kwashiorkor. The child on the right has another type of severe malnutrition, and does not have swelling on the legs or under the eyes.

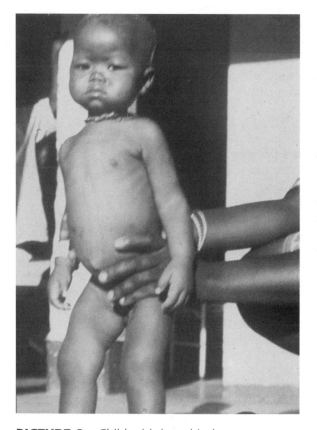

PICTURE 8 *Child with kwashiorkor*

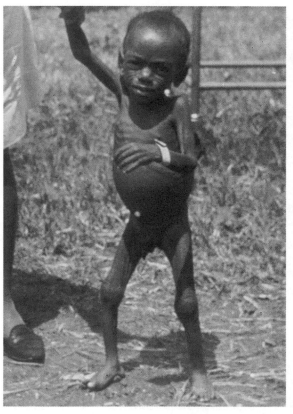

PICTURE 9 *Child with severe malnutrition*

Treating severe malnutrition

Send all children with severe malnutrition to the nutrition clinic. Send children with kwashiorkor to hospital. The nutrition clinic may be in the community or at a hospital.

Children with severe malnutrition usually stay at the clinic for a week or longer.

Tell the students to come and talk to you in the refreshment break if they want to know more about how to run a nutrition clinic. Give them a copy of Appendix 7. This Appendix also describes how to feed children with severe malnutrition.

Refreshment break

SECTION 3: Diagnosis and management of anaemia

Anaemia is a lack of haemoglobin. Haemoglobin is found in red blood cells. Haemoglobin is a protein that contains iron. Anaemia is caused by illnesses that stop the body making haemoglobin or illnesses that damage or waste red blood cells.

Patients with anaemia are weak and are not good at fighting infections. They often have fast breathing. Pregnant women with anaemia may die or give birth to small, weak babies.

Causes of anaemia

POSTER 9:
(Student answer poster)

Causes of anaemia
Divide Poster 9 into two areas. Give one area the title 'Prevent making haemoglobin'. Give the other area the title 'Damage or waste red blood cells'.
Ask the students: What are the most common causes of anaemia in our country?

If sickle cell disease is a problem in your area, teach Appendix 8 at another time.

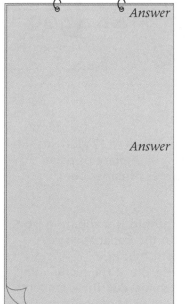

Answer

Answer

*Problems that **prevent** the body **making haemoglobin***
- Patients with **malnutrition** or who **do not eat** a **mixed diet** are not able to make haemoglobin
- **Children** grow very quickly **between** the ages of **6 months and 3 years**. Children should grow very quickly if they are **born very small**. If they do **not** eat foods containing a large amount of **iron** and **folic acid** they will not be able to make haemoglobin

*Problems that **damage or waste red blood cells***
- **Malaria** damages red blood cells
- **Hookworm** cause bleeding into the bowel. A large number of hookworm cause anaemia
- **Pregnancy** uses a lot of iron and folic acid from the woman's body for the baby. If the woman does not eat a mixed diet to replace this iron and folic acid, she will become anaemic. Having many pregnancies in a short time causes anaemia
- Women who **bleed heavily every month** lose a lot of blood (see Lesson 7).
- **Sickle cell disease**.

Activity

| POSTER 10:
(Prepared poster) | **Foods to prevent anaemia**
Copy Picture 10 onto Poster 10. Do *not* draw the circles and triangles on the poster. |

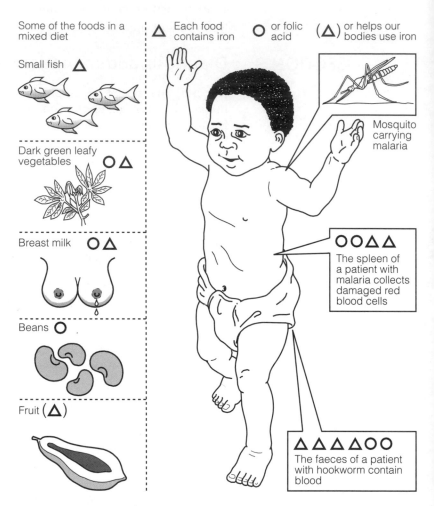

PICTURE 10 *Foods to prevent anaemia*

Give the 10 paper triangles and 7 paper circles to 17 students. Put sticky tape or Blu-tak on the back of each piece of paper or give the students pins to stick the pieces of paper onto Poster 10.

- Explain to the students that **haemoglobin** is made from **iron, folic acid** and protein. Tell them that the paper triangles represent iron and the circles represent folic acid.
- Tell the students that the foods on the left of the picture are examples of foods which prevent anaemia. Ask three students to put a triangle on a food that they think contains **iron**. These

students should put a triangle on the small fish, dark green leafy vegetables and the breastmilk.

- Tell the students that fruit does not contain iron but it contains Vitamin C. **Vitamin C** helps our bodies use the iron in other food. Ask one student to put a triangle on the fruit. Draw brackets ( ) around the triangle.

- Ask three students to put a circle on a food that they think contains **folic acid**. These students should put a circle on the dark green leafy vegetables, the breastmilk and the beans.

If a person or child eats these foods as part of a mixed diet he will be able to make haemoglobin and prevent anaemia. This child eats all of these foods.

Mosquitoes carry malaria. Malaria damages red blood cells and can cause anaemia. The spleen is a rubbish bin for damaged red blood cells. Children who often get malaria may have a large spleen.

- Tell the students that the picture shows a mosquito on the child's skin. Ask four students to put two triangles and two circles near the spleen.

This child also has many hookworm inside his bowel. Hookworm cause bleeding into the bowel. Folic acid and a large amount of iron are lost into the faeces. If a patient has a large number of hookworm in his bowel, he will become anaemic.

- Ask six students to put four triangles and two circles near the faeces.

Preventing anaemia

We can do two things to prevent anaemia:
• help patients to make haemoglobin
• prevent illnesses that damage or waste red blood cells.

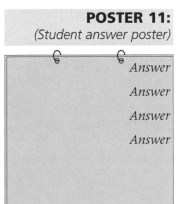

POSTER 11:
(Student answer poster)

Answer

Answer

Answer

Answer

How to prevent anaemia
Ask your students how we can prevent anaemia.

1. Eat a **mixed diet.**

2. **Wear shoes** to **prevent hookworm infections.**

3. Use **latrines.**

4. Use **mosquito nets to prevent malaria**, especially in children under the age of 5 years and pregnant women. Dip nets in permethrin every 6 months or deltamethrin every 12 months. Dip the nets just before the time of year when most people get malaria.

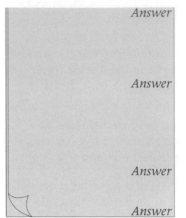

Answer

Answer

Answer

Answer

5. Advise women to wait until their youngest child is 2 years old before having another baby. This helps women to build up a store of folic acid and iron in their bodies. Breastfeeding helps to delay the next pregnancy.

6. Advise women to eat a mixed diet. In areas where iron deficiency is common, give **all pregnant women tablets** of **ferrous sulphate** 200 mg and folic acid 0.4 mg every day (or one tablet of ferrous sulphate 200 mg and one tablet of folic acid 0.25 mg every day).

7. Advise girls to wait until they are at least 17 years old before having a baby.

8. Treat heavy periods (see Lesson 7).

Diagnosing and treating anaemia

Anaemia may have more than one cause. Take the patient's history:

1. Look for general danger signs. Treat serious illnesses like pneumonia immediately.
2. Look for a fever. In malaria areas, treat patients with anaemia, who have a fever, with the first-line malaria treatment immediately.
3. Look for anaemia in the patient's conjunctiva (the inside of the eyelid).
4. Look for fast breathing or fluid under the skin.

   - If the inside of the eyelid looks less red than usual, or you cannot see the lines on the palm of the hand, the patient has anaemia.
   - If the patient also has fast breathing or fluid under the skin, he may have severe anaemia. Give him the first-line malaria treatment if there is malaria in the area. Send him to hospital immediately.
   - If a patient with anaemia does not have fast breathing or swollen legs, the patient has moderate anaemia. Treat patients with moderate anaemia with ferrous sulphate for 3 months if possible.
   - If a woman with moderate anaemia is pregnant, measure her haemoglobin or send her to hospital. If her haemoglobin is less than 7 g/dl give her the first-line malaria treatment and send her to hospital.

POSTER 12:
(Prepared poster)

How to treat anaemia
Copy Table 3 onto Poster 12.

TABLE 3 How to treat anaemia

Priority	Illness	Treatment
1	*Malaria*, in malaria areas, **if the patient has a fever**	**If the first-line malaria treatment is chloroquine:** *Chloroquine for 3 days. Give advice about tepid sponging. Return after finishing the medicine for further treatment.*
1	*Malaria*, in malaria areas, **if the patient has a fever**	**If the first-line malaria treat ment is Fansidar:** *Fansidar at health centre. Give advice about tepid sponging. Also treat and give advice about hookworm. Return after finishing the medicine for further treatment.*
2	**Hookworm**	Ask if the patient may be pregnant. Mebendazole for 3 days. Do not give mebendazole to patients less than 1 year old or women in the first 3 months of pregnancy. Give patients advice about wearing shoes and using latrines. Return after finishing the medicine for further treatment.
3	**Poor diet**	Ferrous sulphate for 3 months if possible. Give advice about eating a mixed diet.
4	**Other causes of anaemia**	Treat the cause. The patient may be pregnant, have heavy periods or an infection that goes on for a long time.
5	*Frequent malaria*	*If a patient continues to have anaemia after 3 months, examine the abdomen. If you can feel the spleen, give the patient medicine to prevent malaria and ferrous sulphate (at the lower dose) for 3 months.*

Table 4 summarises the doses of ferrous sulphate to use to treat anaemia. If you do not have enough ferrous sulphate, give a lower dose for 3 months.

<table>
<tr><td>**POSTER 13:**
(Prepared poster)</td></tr>
</table>

POSTER 13:
(Prepared poster)

Doses of ferrous sulphate
Copy Table 4 onto Poster 13.

TABLE 4 Doses of ferrous sulphate

Patient's weight	Dose of ferrous sulphate to treat anaemia (200 mg tablets) for 3 months	
	Best dose	**Lower dose**
15 kg or less	$\frac{1}{4}$ tablet 2 times a day	$\frac{1}{4}$ tablet 1 time a day
16–29 kg	$\frac{1}{2}$ tablet 2 times a day	$\frac{1}{2}$ tablet 1 time a day
30–44 kg	1 tablet 2 times a day	1 tablet 1 time a day
45 kg and above	1 tablet 3 times a day	1 tablet 1 time a day

SECTION 4:   When to send patients to hospital

Give each student a copy of Appendix 6. Make sure that the students know how to use Appendix 6.

Ask your students which patients we should send to a hospital or a nutrition clinic. Look for the following answers:

Answer   Children with fluid under the skin

Answer   Children with a growth line that has gone down at the two most recent weighings

Answer   Patients (including pregnant women) with very pale conjunctivae and fast breathing or fluid under the skin

Answer   Pregnant women with a haemoglobin of less than 7 g/dl

Lunch break

SECTION 5:   Practical

Tell the students that the four role plays will help them practise diagnosis and treatment of malnutrition or anaemia. Divide the class into six groups, with at least three students in each group. In each group, one student will play the doctor, one student will play the patient or the patient's mother, and a third student will be the observer. For each role play:

- Give the patient (or patient's mother) a piece of paper which describes the patient's symptoms and what food he normally eats. If the doctor asks the correct questions, the patient will tell the doctor what symptoms he has and what he normally eats.
- Give the patient's mother the appropriate growth chart if the patient is less than 5 years old.
- Give the doctor a piece of paper which tells the doctor what she will find when she examines the patient. The doctor will find out the patient's age and take the patient's history. The doctor will look at the growth chart. She will also use Appendix 6 to decide what the diagnosis and treatment are.
- Give the observer a piece of paper. This piece of paper tells the observer: (1) The diagnosis, (2) The treatment, (3) Advice for the patient, and (4) Whether the patient should be sent to hospital. After each role play the observer will tell the group what the doctor did correctly and what the doctor could have done better.

Role plays

Tell the students that they have 30 minutes to do the first three of the four role plays. A different student should pretend to be the doctor, patient and observer in each role play. Tell them to use Appendix 6. Stop the activity after the third role play.

- Give each group the four role plays.

ROLE PLAY 1:

You are the **mother** of a 15-month-old child, Sunday Otala. You are pregnant again. You stopped breastfeeding your child a week ago because you think that breastfeeding will harm the unborn baby. You feed the child two times a day, normally rice, maize meal or bread.

You are the **doctor**. You see that the child's conjunctivae are not pale. He does not look unwell but he is crying. There is no fluid under the skin. Ask to look at the growth chart (Picture 11).

You are the **observer**. The child has early malnutrition. The doctor should take a quick but good history. The doctor should give mebendazole and advise the mother to follow the six rules of good nutrition. The doctor should also advise the mother to start breastfeeding again immediately. Breastfeeding will not harm either the unborn child or the patient.

ROLE PLAY 2:

You are the **patient**. You are a mother aged 28 years. You are 5 months pregnant. You feel dizzy and you have a headache.

You are the **doctor**. You see that the woman's conjunctivae are pale. She does not have a fever. The patient has a swelling in her abdomen which is the correct size for a 5-month pregnancy. She breathes less than 25 times in a minute and she does not have swollen ankles. You measure her haemoglobin. Her haemoglobin is 8 g/dl.

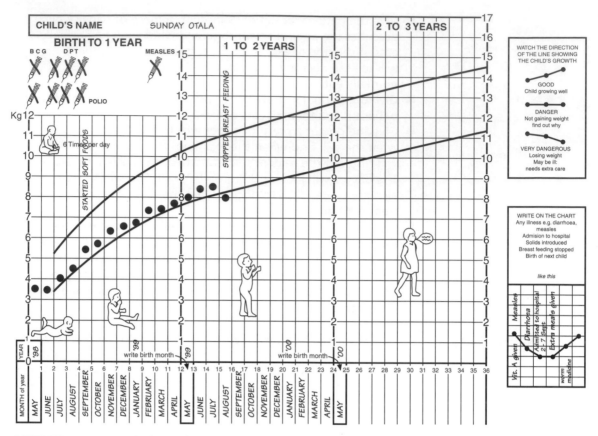

PICTURE 11 *Growth chart of child in role play 1*

You are the **observer**. The patient has anaemia. She does not have a fever. She does not need treatment for malaria. The doctor should treat and give advice for hookworm. The doctor should also ask the woman to come back to the health centre after finishing the hookworm medicine. On the next visit, the doctor should advise a mixed diet and give ferrous sulphate until she gives birth.

ROLE PLAY 3: You are the **mother** of a 3-year-old child, Tunji Kehinde. You do not think that your child has a problem. The child has diarrhoea often. You feed the child three times a day with cassava, maize meal… 'all the usual foods'.

You are the **doctor**. The conjunctivae are not pale. The child does not smile and has no interest in what is going on around him. The child's legs are swollen. After you press the leg with your finger for 10 seconds, you can see where you were pressing. Ask to look at his growth chart (Picture 12).

You are the **observer**. The child has kwashiorkor. The doctor should send him to hospital immediately.

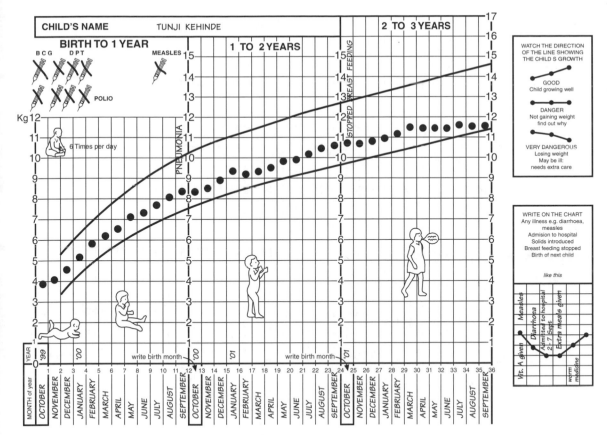

PICTURE 12 *Growth chart of child in role play 3*

If you do not use direct recording scales in your country, cross out the following box and fill in the last two weights on the growth chart in Picture 13. The last two weights have gone down.

Tell your students that each group in turn will now fill in the last two weights using the direct recording scale. Replace the sling under the direct recording scale with a bucket. (The bucket represents the child being weighed.)

Each group should partly fill the bucket with enough water so that the pointer of the direct recording scale lies over the last weight. Move the scale forward one month. Remove a cupful of water from the bucket. Do not throw this water away. Ask a student to mark the 'child's' new weight. Ask a student to move the scale forward and remove another cupful of water. Ask another student to mark the next weight. Remove the growth chart and allow the group to do the last role play. (Replace the water in the bucket ready for the next group of students.)

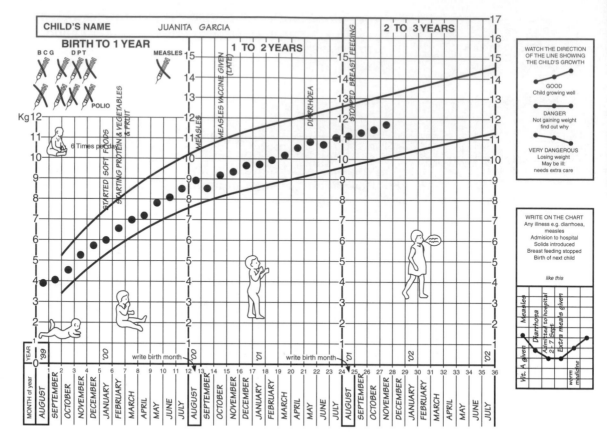

PICTURE 13 *Growth chart of child in role play 4*

ROLE PLAY 4:	You are the **mother** of a 2½-year-old girl, Juanita Garcia Lopez. The girl has had a fever for 3 days. You feed her rice, cassava, maize porridge and occasionally small fish two times a day.

You are the **doctor**. The conjunctivae are not pale. The child does not smile. The child does not have swollen legs. You look at her growth chart (Picture 13). The growth line has gone down on the two most recent weighings.

You are the **observer**. The child may have severe malnutrition. The doctor should send the child to a nutrition clinic.

SECTION 7:   Answers to the quiz

Ask the students to call out the answers to each question in the quiz.

1. What do the following growth lines mean? What will you do for each child? (Refer to the illustrations of the growth lines in the quiz at the beginning of this chapter.)

   • **The child is growing well. Tell the mother that the child is growing well.**

- **The child is not growing. Take the child's history. Treat any illness. Teach the mother the six rules of good nutrition.**
- **The child has lost weight. Treat for early malnutrition. If the child has lost weight on the two most recent weighings, send him to the nutrition clinic.**

2. What are the six rules of good nutrition?
   - **Breastfeed until second birthday at least six times a day.**
   - **Soft foods in addition to breastmilk after 5 months.**
   - **Protein foods in addition to breastmilk after 6 months.**
   - **Vitamin and mineral foods in addition to breastmilk after 6 months.**
   - **Four meals a day in addition to breastmilk after 9 months.**
   - **If ill, feed more often. Breastfeed young babies eight times a day or feed five times a day.**

3. What will happen if a child is not given food which follows the six rules of good nutrition?
   - **The child may get malnutrition or anaemia. He may get severe malnutrition. Many patients with severe malnutrition die.**

4. What are the causes of anaemia?
   - **Malnutrition – lack of iron and folic acid in the diet**
   - **Malaria**
   - **Hookworm**
   - **Frequent pregnancy**
   - **Sickle cell disease**
   - **Heavy periods – women who bleed heavily every month lose a lot of blood.**

Lesson 5   Skin problems

BEFORE THE LESSON

■ There are 11 posters in this lesson. (See p. 4 for information on how to use the posters.)
Prepared posters: 1
Student answer posters: 2, 4, 7, 8, 10
Summary posters: 3, 5, 6, 9, 11

■ For section 2, you need four patients. You need one patient with a fungus infection, one with impetigo, one with scabies and one with a skin ulcer.

■ Ask the patients to meet you in the classroom at 8:30 a.m. Tell them that they will receive a small payment for coming. Do not forget to bring some money with you to the lesson.

■ Prepare *blank* copies of the five tables under 'Features of skin problems' for each student. Copy the headings only and leave the boxes empty.

■ You need a balloon filled with water.

■ You need a copy of Appendix 9 for each student.

■ You need six copies of the patient case study questions for the practical in section 4.

SECTION 1:   Quiz

POSTER 1:
(Prepared poster)

Quiz
Ask the students to answer the questions on their own. Do not give the answers until the end of the lesson.

> 1. For which skin problem would you use each of the following medicines?
>   Benzyl benzoate emulsion
>   Whitfield ointment
>   Co-trimoxazole
>   Gentian violet
>
> 2. How do you diagnose measles?
>
> 3. If a patient has new dark red spots in the skin, what should you do?

SECTION 2:   Diagnosis and management of skin problems

Give each of your students one blank copy of Tables 1 to 5 (see pp. 79–82). Students should complete their blank tables with the correct answers after each problem has been discussed. If possible, show the students each important feature on a patient.

POSTER 2:
(Student answer poster)

Features of skin problems – Virus infections

Draw the *lines and headings only* of Table 1 (on p. 79) on Poster 2.

Today we will learn about skin problems that are caused by:
• virus infections
• bacterial infections
• fungus infection
• insects
• allergies.

For each skin problem, we will fill in the appropriate table. You can put the finished tables on your health centre wall.

Virus infections

Three viruses that can cause a skin rash or swelling are:
• measles
• chickenpox
• warts.

Measles

Measles starts with a runny nose, sticky eyes, a fever and a cough. A few days later a flat red rash appears behind the ears. Next, the rash becomes slightly raised and spreads to the face and body. The areas of redness meet together. The rash lasts for 6 or 7 days. The rash does not itch. The fever disappears soon after the rash has appeared, usually within 3 days. The patient may also have red eyes.

If a patient has a fever and a rash all over his body, he may have measles. The rash does not itch. Diagnose measles if the patient also has red eyes or a cough or fluid coming from the nose.

Treat a patient with measles as described in Lesson 3:
• Look for chest illnesses.
• Look for corneal ulcers.
• Do not give tetracycline eye ointment for conjunctivitis unless a cornea is not clear.
• Give vitamin A.
• Give the first-line malaria treatment if there is malaria in your area.
• Show the mother how to do tepid sponging.
• Advise the mother to continue to breastfeed.
• Advise the mother to give a mixed diet of mashed food five times each day. She should do this until the child is well again and for a week after he is better.

Ask the students what to write in each space of the measles row of Table 1. Fill in the correct answers on Poster 2. Students should fill in the correct answers in their blank Table 1.

Chickenpox

The first symptoms of chickenpox are a rash and a fever. The rash quickly turns into small blisters on the body and under the hair. Next, blisters appear on the face, arms and legs. The blisters are very itchy. Many patients scratch the blisters and damage the skin. This can cause impetigo (infection with bacteria). Treat impetigo if it is bigger than 1 cm wide.

POSTER 3:
(Summary poster)

Advice for patients with chickenpox

1. **Cut** your **fingernails**. Long fingernails damage the skin if the patient scratches her skin.

2. **Wash** frequently to prevent impetigo.

3. **Give home treatment advice**.
   - Give plenty of **fluids**.
   - Continue to **feed** at least **five times a day**.
   - Tell the patient to **return**:
     - **if** she is **not able to drink**
     - **if** her **breathing** becomes **difficult or fast**
     - **if** she becomes **more ill**.

Now ask the students what to write in each space of the chickenpox row of Table 1. Fill in the correct answers on Poster 2. Students should fill in the correct answers in their blank Table 1.

Warts

The wart virus causes warts on the skin, often on the hands or feet. Warts are normally the same colour as the skin. They are often raised above the surrounding skin. Warts do not itch. It may take months or years for warts to disappear but warts do not need any treatment.

Ask the students what to write in each space of the warts row of Table 1. Fill in the correct answers on Poster 2. Students should fill in the correct answers in their blank Table 1.

POSTER 4:
(Student answer poster)

Features of skin problems – Bacterial infections
Draw the *lines and headings only* of Table 2 (on pp. 80–81) on Poster 4.

Bacterial infections

Bacterial infections that can affect the skin are:
- impetigo
- skin ulcers
- abscess
- meningococcal septicaemia
- serious skin infections in children less than 2 months old.

Impetigo

Impetigo starts as a blister that quickly gets bigger and breaks. The skin becomes wet and red and dries to form a yellow coloured area. Impetigo is most common on the face, hands and feet. People get impetigo by touching the skin of a person who has impetigo. A person is more likely to get impetigo if he has scabies, flea bites or does not wash often.

Impetigo does not cause a fever and is not painful. If the area underneath the skin becomes infected, the patient has cellulitis. A patient with cellulitis may have a fever and the skin is painful to touch.

Treat a patient with impetigo as follows:
- If the impetigo is smaller than 10 cm wide, paint it with gentian violet once a day for 5 days.
- If the impetigo is bigger than 10 cm wide, treat with co-trimoxazole, at the normal dose, for 5 days.
- If there is cellulitis, give co-trimoxazole, at the normal dose, for 5 days.

Advise a patient with impetigo to:
1. Cut his fingernails.
2. Come back if his skin becomes more painful or he develops a fever.
3. Wash every day and to eat a mixed diet.

Ask the students what to write in each space of the impetigo row of Table 2. Fill in the correct answers on Poster 4. Students should fill in the correct answers in their blank Table 2.

Skin ulcers

If a skin wound does not heal, a skin ulcer develops. Bacteria in the wound, malnutrition or diabetes may stop a wound from healing. Patients with leprosy may have many wounds and skin ulcers. Skin ulcers are normally on the feet and ankles.

POSTER 5:
(Summary poster)

How to treat skin ulcers

Treat skin ulcers like this:
1. **Wash** the ulcer **every day** if possible.

2. On the **first visit**:
   - Clean the ulcer. Squirt **normal saline or clean water** quickly at the ulcer **using** a **syringe**.

(*continued*)
- Do this again and again until all the dirt has been removed.
- Next, put **polyvidone iodine on the ulcer**.

3. On the second visit, and **further visits**:
   - Clean the ulcer very gently. Do not damage the healing red skin.
   - **Gently** remove the yellow or green matter from the ulcer using a sterile swab or cloth. Dip the cloth in **normal saline or polyvodine iodine** 10%.

4. **Cover** the ulcer each day with a clean dressing. Use unripe slices of **papaya** flesh underneath the dressing bandage as an antiseptic if possible. Otherwise use polyvidone iodine 10%.

5. **If** the skin around the ulcer is **painful** to touch, the patient has **cellulitis**. Treat the patient with co-trimoxazole, at the normal dose, for 5 days.

6. Make sure that the patient has been immunised against tetanus. If she has not, give a **tetanus toxoid vaccination** this week. Give two more tetanus toxoid vaccinations, with a month between each injection. This will not prevent the patient from getting tetanus from the ulcer she has now, but it will prevent tetanus in future. The vaccine starts to work after 3 months and gives protection for 10 years or more.

7. **If** a skin ulcer is **no better after 2 weeks** of treatment, send the patient to **hospital**. The patient may need treatment for another cause of the ulcer, for example diabetes, malnutrition or cutaneous leishmaniasis. The edges of a cutaneous leishmaniasis ulcer are raised.

Now ask the students what to write in each space of the skin ulcers row of Table 2. Fill in the correct answers on Poster 4. Students should fill in the correct answers in their blank Table 2.

Abscess

An abscess is a type of bacterial infection underneath the skin. The body uses white blood cells to fight against the infection. Dead white blood cells collect to make a lump filled with yellow matter called pus. An abscess is warm and painful when you touch it. It often feels like a balloon that is full of fluid.

Use a balloon filled with water to show your students what it feels like to touch an abscess. Ask the students to place two fingers on the balloon and to press one of the fingers down into the balloon. The balloon pushes the second finger upwards.

Women who are breastfeeding often get an abscess in a breast. Breast abscesses develop if the baby does not take the nipple all the way into the mouth when he is breastfeeding. This damages the skin of the nipple. Bacteria can get into the damaged skin and may cause an abscess.

POSTER 6:
(Summary poster)

How to treat an abscess

Treat an abscess as follows:

1. Cut into the abscess with a **sterile knife**.

2. Clean the pus out of the abscess.

3. Put a **sterile swab**, which has been dipped **in normal saline or polyvidone iodine** 10%, as far **into the hole** as possible.

4. Leave a new sterile swab in the opening of the hole.

5. The wound will heal from the inside. Keep the hole open, this will allow you to clean the inside of the wound.

6. Treat the patient with **co-trimoxazole**, at the normal dose, for 5 days.

7. Gently **remove** all of the **swabs** from the wound **every second day**. Put new sterile swabs back in.

If the abscess is in a breast:

1. Make the cut in a line pointing away from the nipple.

2. Express breastmilk frequently from that breast, every 4 hours, by holding the breast firmly and gently squeezing the nipple between the thumb and a finger.

3. Use a cup and spoon to give the milk to the baby. Do not give the milk if it has a lot of pus in it.
   • If a breast is hot and painful to touch but does not yet feel like a balloon, put a large needle into the lump. Pull the plunger of the syringe: if pus comes out, make a cut in the breast.
   • If there is no pus, give the woman co-trimoxazole at the normal dose. See the woman again after 2 days.

Now ask the students what to write in each space of the abscess row of Table 2. Fill in the correct answers on Poster 4. Students should fill in the correct answers in their blank Table 2.

Meningococcal septicaemia

We will talk about meningococcal septicaemia later in this lesson. Leave space in your blank Table 2.

Serious skin infections in children less than 2 months old

Young babies can become ill and die very quickly. Young babies with serious infections may not always have a general danger sign. Look for a fever. Look at the skin and at the umbilicus in the middle of the baby's abdomen.

If the young baby has:
- pus coming from the umbilicus or redness of the umbilicus *and* a fever
- many or large areas of pus under the skin,

give him an intramuscular injection of chloramphenicol. Give 40 mg (0.2 ml) for each kg of body weight. Send him to hospital immediately.

If the young baby has:
- pus coming from the umbilicus, but no fever
- redness of the umbilicus, but no fever
- only small areas of pus under the skin,

give him co-trimoxazole, ½ tablet two times a day, for 5 days. See the child again after 2 days.

Ask the students what to write in each space of the row for serious skin infections in children less than 2 months old in Table 2. Fill in the correct answers on Poster 4. Students should fill in the correct answers in their blank Table 2.

Fungus infections

POSTER 7:
(Student answer poster)

Features of skin problems – Fungus infections
Draw the *lines and headings only* of Table 3 (p. 81) on Poster 7.

Fungus infections that affect the skin are:
- tinea
- yeast infections.

Tinea

Tinea is a fungus infection. It can grow anywhere on the skin. Tinea starts as a scaly, slightly raised pale or red patch. The skin is not painful when you touch it. The rash may be itchy. As the infection grows, the skin in the middle of the rash may become normal again. The infection then looks like a ring. Tinea causes hairs to fall out of the skin. Treating tinea takes a long time. The medicine you use will depend on what is available locally.
- Rub Whitfield ointment (benzoic acid and salicylic acid ointment) into the skin once a day for several weeks. Advise the patient to continue using the ointment until the rash has completely disappeared and for one extra week.
- If the problem is no better after 4 weeks, send the patient to the leprosy clinic. Leprosy can also cause the skin to look pale and scaly.
- If the tinea is in the hair, skin treatments will not help.

Give the students a copy of Appendix 9.

Ask the students what to write in each space of the tinea row in Table 3. Fill in the correct answers on Poster 7. Students should fill in the correct answers in their blank Table 3.

Yeast infections

Yeasts are a special type of fungus. Yeasts grow in warm, wet areas of the body. Yeast infections are found between the toes, near the private parts, under the breasts and under the arms. The skin will be slightly wet. The skin may be white or red.

Treat yeast infections with gentian violet or a fungus treatment. Give this every day until the rash has completely disappeared, and for one extra week after that.

Ask the students what to write in each space of the yeasts row in Table 3. Fill in the correct answers on Poster 7. Students should fill in the correct answers in their blank Table 3.

Insects

POSTER 8:
(Student answer poster)

Features of skin problems: Insect problems
Draw the *lines and headings only* of Table 4 (p. 81) on Poster 8.

Skin problems caused by insects are:
• flea bites
• body lice infestation
• scabies.

Flea bites

Fleas live in the homes and clothes of people and on animals. Flea bites are itchy. If people scratch the bites, this can damage the skin and cause impetigo. Advise patients with flea bites to clean their home. Tell them to put insecticide powder on floors, bedding and clothes, if possible.

Ask the students what to write in each space of the flea bites row in Table 4. Fill in the correct answers on Poster 8. Students should fill in the correct answers in their blank Table 4.

Body lice infestation

Body lice live in people's clothes. Body lice cause an itchy rash on most parts of the body. This rash is similar to the itchy rash caused by scabies. Treat the skin with benzyl benzoate emulsion. Advise the patient to wash his clothes in very hot water and to iron the clothes to kill the lice.

Ask the students what to write in each space of the body lice row in Table 4. Fill in the correct answers on Poster 8. Students should fill in the correct answers in their blank Table 4.

Scabies

Scabies is very common. It is caused by a tiny insect that lives underneath the skin. A patient with scabies has scaly skin, often at the wrists or between his fingers. He may have an itchy rash over most of his body. Treat the skin with benzyl benzoate emulsion. Advise the patient to wash his clothes in very hot water and to iron the clothes.

A person with scabies may get impetigo. If he has impetigo, treat this before using benzyl benzoate emulsion to treat the scabies. Tell the patient to cut his fingernails.

POSTER 9:
(Summary poster)

How to treat scabies

Treat scabies as follows:
- Treat **everyone in the house**. Some people have scabies without having symptoms.
- Use one **100 ml** bottle of **benzyl benzoate** (25%) **to treat two adults** or children over the age of 5 years.
- If the patient is **under the age of 2 years mix** the benzyl benzoate **with** an **equal amount of water**.
- Put benzyl benzoate on all parts of the body, except for the face and head.
- **Leave** the medicine on for **24 hours**.
- **Repeat** this treatment **after 7 days**.
- Treatment will kill all the scabies insects, but the skin will still itch for up to 2 weeks.
- If the rash is no better 3 weeks after treating the whole family, there may be another cause of the skin rash. In areas where there is river blindness, the rash may be caused by onchocerciasis. Treat everyone with ivermectin 6 mg once a year. This will help to prevent blindness but it will not help the skin rash.

Ask the students what to write in each space of the scabies row in Table 4. Fill in the correct answers on Poster 8. Students should fill in the correct answers in their blank Table 4.

Allergy problems

POSTER 10:
(Student answer poster)

Features of skin problems – Allergy problems
Draw the *lines and headings only* of Table 5 (p. 82) on Poster 10.

Allergy problems that can cause a skin rash are:
- reactions to medicines
- eczema.

Reactions to medicines

Injections, tablets or ointments can cause skin rashes. Antibiotics and phenobarbital commonly cause rashes. Allergic rashes are often itchy, but are not usually scaly. If a rash starts or gets worse after using any medicine, stop the medicine immediately.

Ask the students what to write in each space of the reactions to medicines row in Table 5. Fill in the correct answers on Poster 10. Students should fill in the correct answers in their blank Table 5.

Eczema

An eczema rash is itchy and scaly. Eczema often causes a rash at the front of the elbows, behind the knees, and on the face. It also causes dry skin.

Eczema is difficult to treat. Tell the patient that you will not be able to cure eczema. To treat skin dryness, put natural oils, such as coconut oil, on the skin **every** day. Tell the patient not to use perfumed soap and to avoid using soap frequently. Soap removes oils from the skin. If the eczema is very itchy, put hydrocortisone cream 1% on the affected areas two times a day until the itch is better.

Ask the students what to write in each space of the eczema row in Table 5. Fill in the correct answers on Poster 10. Students should fill in the correct answers in their blank Table 5.

Tables 1–5: Features of skin problems

TABLE 1   Features of skin problems – Virus infections

	Rash	Where	Other features	Sometimes	Advice	Treatment
Measles	1. Flat then slightly raised 2. Red 3. Does **not** itch	Starts behind ears Goes to face and body Goes to all parts of the body	Fever Has one of: (a) cough (b) conjunctivitis (c) fluid from the nose	1. Pneumonia 2. Corneal ulcer	Home treatment Breastfeed Soft mixed diet 5 times a day Tepid sponge	Vitamin A The first-line malaria treatment in malaria areas Send to hospital if has pneumonia
Chickenpox	1. Itchy 2. Blisters	Starts on body and in hair Goes to arms and legs	Fever	Impetigo	Cut nails Wash daily Home treatment	The first-line malaria treatment in malaria areas No other medicine Treat if has impetigo

TABLE 1 (*continued*)

	Rash	Where	Other features	Sometimes	Advice	Treatment
Warts	1. No colour 2. Raised 3. Not itchy 4. Hard and dry	Hands or feet	None		Warts will go away after several months or years	None

TABLE 2 Features of skin problems – Bacteria infections

	Rash	Where	Other features	Sometimes	Advice	Treatment
Impetigo	Blisters, then wet red skin, then dry yellow matter	Face, hands or feet	None	Cellulitis	Cut nails Wash daily Home treatment Return if develops fever or pain	Gentian violet if less than 10 cm Co-trimoxazole if more than 10 cm Co-trimoxazole if tender
Skin ulcers	1. Skin broken 2. Red, yellow or green matter in wound	Ankles and feet	None	Cellulitis	Keep dry and change dressing daily	Wash and dress everyday. Use polyvidone iodine or unripe papaya under dressing Tetanus vaccine Treat if has cellulitis
Abscess	1. Hot and painful to touch 2. Feels like a balloon	Breast or anywhere	Fever		Come to health centre every second day Express breastmilk and give to child with cup and spoon	Cut and clean Co-trimoxazole
Meningo-cocal septicaemia	Dark red spots that do not disappear when pressed	Anywhere	Unwell, often a general danger sign			Intramuscular benzylpenicillin and send to hospital immediately

TABLE 2 (*continued*)

	Rash	Where	Other features	Sometimes	Advice	Treatment
Serious skin infections in child less than 2 months	1. Pus or red umbilicus **and** fever OR 2, many or large areas of pus under skin	Anywhere, often umbilicus	Fever or any general danger sign			Intramuscular chloramphenicol. Send to hospital immediately

TABLE 3 Features of skin problems – Fungus infections

	Rash	Where	Other features	Sometimes	Advice	Treatment
Tinea	1. Scaly 2. Slightly raised	Anywhere	None		Go to leprosy clinic if no better after 4 weeks	Whitfield ointment or other treatment for fungus
Yeasts	1. Wet 2. Itchy	Between fingers, toes, under breasts, armpits and next to private parts				Gentian violet or treatment for fungus

TABLE 4 Features of skin problems – Insect problems

	Rash	Where	Other features	Sometimes	Advice	Treatment
Flea bites	Itchy spots	Anywhere		Impetigo	Clean home. Insecticide dust on floors, bedding and clothes	None
Body lice	Itchy rash	All parts of body			Wash clothes in very hot water and use hot iron How to use benzyl benzoate	Benzyl benzoate emulsion for whole family
Scabies	1. Scaly 2. Itchy	Wrists Between fingers Anywhere but not face or scalp	Itchy rash on all parts of body	Impetigo	Cut nails How to use benzyl benzoate Return if no better after 3 weeks	Benzyl benzoate for whole family

TABLE 5 Features of skin problems – Allergy

	Rash	Where	Other features	Sometimes	Advice	Treatment
Reaction to medicine	1. Often itchy 2. Dark or red 3. Often blisters	One area, all of the body		Anaphylaxis and death	Stop medicine	Treat anaphylaxis
Eczema	1. Itchy 2. Scaly	Front of elbows, behind the knees, neck and face			Use coconut oil every day Do not use perfumed soap	1% hydrocortisone cream

Refreshment break

SECTION 3: When to send patients to hospital

POSTER 11:
(Prepared poster)

When to send patients with skin problems to hospital

Send patients with skin problems to hospital **immediately if**:

1. They have **pneumonia and measles**. Give patients with pneumonia and measles an intramuscular injection of procaine penicillin fortified (0.1 million IU for each kg of body weight up to 1.2 million IU, one time). Pneumonia is very dangerous to patients who have measles.

2. They have **meningococcal septicaemia**. If a patient has new, dark red spots in the skin, press on the spots with two fingers. Separate the two fingers. If the **dark red spots do not disappear when you press** on the spots, treat the patient for meningococcal septicaemia. Give her an intramuscular injection of benzylpenicillin (0.1 million IU for each kg of body weight, up to 2 million IU, one time). If the patient is not able to get to the hospital immediately, give benzylpenicillin four times a day.

Show the students how to press on the spots with two fingers. Ask the students what to write in each space of the meningococcal septicaemia row of Table 2.

3. A **serious skin infection** in a **child aged less than 2 months**. Give the child an intramuscular injection of chloramphenicol (40 mg for each kg of body weight one time).

Also send these patients to hospital:
- If a skin ulcer is no better after 2 weeks of treatment. The patient may have diabetes, malnutrition or cutaneous leishmaniasis.
- If a rash is no better after 4 weeks of treatment with a fungus treatment, send him to the leprosy clinic.

SECTION 4:   Practical

Activity   Divide the students into three groups. Give two copies of the following patient case studies to each group. Tell the students that they will use their five tables of the features of skin problems to decide which skin problem each patient has.

Using the tables, they should:
- make sure that the *rash* is the correct type
- check *where* the rash is
- see what *other features* the patient has.

Tell the students that they have 15 minutes to answer the questions about three patients. If the type of rash, the location of the rash and other features are correct, they have made the diagnosis.

Patient 1   A 4-year-old girl has an itchy rash on her body and in her hair. The girl has a slight fever. She does not have a cough or difficult breathing. Her eyes look normal. Some areas of skin have blisters.
1. What skin problem does she have?
2. What other illness may she have?
3. What is the correct treatment?

Patient 2   A 35-year-old woman complains of swelling and pain in her left breast. She has a 2-month-old baby. The woman has a fever and a hot swelling on her left breast. The skin is painful and feels like a balloon when you touch it.
1. What skin problem does she have?
2. What treatment would you give her?
3. What advice will you give her?

Patient 3   An 11-year-old boy fell on some rocks 2 days ago. The boy has an ulcer on his left shin which looks very dirty.
1. What will you do?
2. He comes back to your health centre 7 days later. When you touch the skin on his left shin, he tells you that it is painful. How will you treat him?

Ask a different student in each group to tell you the answers for each patient. Tell the students what was good about their answers. Tell the students the correct answers. The correct answers are below:

Answers

Patient 1

1. Chickenpox
2. Possibly malaria
3. Give the girl the first-line malaria treatment in malaria areas. Cut her fingernails. Advise her mother to wash her daily. Give the mother advice about home treatment.

Patient 2

1. Breast abscess.
2. Cut into the abscess and clean it. Treat the woman with co-trimoxazole, 2 tablets two times a day, for 5 days.
3. Advise her to express breastmilk and give it to the child with a cup and spoon.

Patient 3

1. Wash and dress the ulcer every day. Use polyvidone iodine or unripe papaya under the dressing. Make sure that the patient has already been immunised against tetanus. If not, give him a tetanus toxoid vaccination this week. Give two more tetanus toxoid vaccinations, with a month between each injection.
2. The boy has cellulitis, give him co-trimoxazole, at the normal dose, for 5 days.

SECTION 5: Answers to the quiz

Ask the students to call out the answers to each question in the quiz.

1. For which skin problem would you use each of the following medicines?
   Benzyl benzoate emulsion
   Scabies
   Whitfield ointment (benzoic acid and salicylic acid ointment)
   Tinea or yeast infection
   Co-trimoxazole
   Cellulitis
   Abscess, after making a cut
   Impetigo, if the area affected is more than 10 cm wide
   Gentian violet
   Yeast infections, impetigo (if the area affected is less than 10 cm wide)

2. How do you diagnose measles?
   Think of measles if a patient has a fever and a rash all over his body. The rash does not itch. Diagnose measles if the patient also has red eyes or a cough or fluid coming from the nose.

3. If a patient has new dark red spots in the skin what should you do?
   Press on the spots with two fingers. Separate the two fingers. If the dark red spots do not disappear, when you press on them, treat the patient for meningococcal septicaemia. Give her an intramuscular injection of benzylpenicillin. Send the patient to hospital immediately.

Lesson 6   Diarrhoea

BEFORE THE LESSON

- There are six posters in this lesson. (See p. 4 for information on how to use the posters.)
  Prepared poster: 1, 3, 4, 5
  Student answer posters: 2, 6

- Ask one student to help you with the demonstration tutorial in this lesson. Give the student a copy of Appendix 10. If possible, practise with him before the lesson.

- Ask a different student to volunteer to teach the class. Make a copy of the 'Demonstration – What to teach village leaders' on page 90 and give it to the volunteer student. Ask her to practise with you before the lesson.

- Give each student a copy of Appendix 10.

- Prepare copies of the role plays. Write the information for the patient, the doctor and the observer on separate pieces of paper. Use a paper clip to keep each role play together. You need one copy each for six groups of students.

- Give each student a copy of Appendices 11 and 12.

- If there is polio in your area, give each student a copy of Appendix 13.

SECTION 1:   Quiz

POSTER 1:
(Prepared poster)

Quiz
Ask the students to answer the questions on their own. Do not give the answers until the end of the lesson.

1. When should you use antibiotics to treat patients who have diarrhoea?

2. What are the causes of diarrhoea?

3. How can you tell if a patient is dehydrated?

4. When should patients with diarrhoea be sent to hospital?

SECTION 2:   Diagnosis and management

A patient with diarrhoea passes loose or watery faeces three or more times in a day. Diarrhoea is dangerous because loose or watery faeces contain a lot of water. If a patient loses a lot of water, he may become dehydrated and may die. Diarrhoea is most common in children aged between 6 months and 18 months. Diarrhoea often kills these children.

Causes of diarrhoea

Tell the students that today they will learn how to prevent and treat diarrhoea.

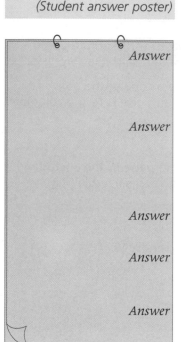

Causes of diarrhoea

Ask the students what causes diarrhoea.

Answer **Bad hygiene – bad hygiene** allows the infections which cause **gastroenteritis** to pass from one person to another person. Gastroenteritis is an infection with bacteria, viruses or parasites which causes diarrhoea.

Answer Bacteria – some **bacteria grow in food** that has been left for a long time before eating. These bacteria cause **food poisoning**. Food poisoning often causes vomiting and/or diarrhoea. If food has been left for 8 hours or more, cook it again. Boil the food for at least 5 minutes.

Answer **Malnutrition** makes a patient more likely to get infections that cause diarrhoea.

Answer Any illness which causes a **fever**, for example malaria, pneumonia, tonsillitis, measles and otitis media can cause diarrhoea.

Answer Any **severe illness**, for example appendicitis and intussusception, can cause diarrhoea. Make sure that patients with diarrhoea do not have peritonitis.

Taking a history and examination

Give each student a copy of Appendix 10. Give a copy of the demonstration to the student who will help you with the demonstration. Ask him to play the part of a student. You will play the student's trainer. Read to the class slowly and in a loud voice. Ask the class to watch and listen to the demonstration.

Four questions for patients with diarrhoea
Copy the four questions from the boxes on p. 87 onto Poster 3.

Demonstration

Student: *What should I do when I see a patient with diarrhoea?*

Trainer: Appendix 10 will help you treat patients with diarrhoea. Start at the top left. The treatment for diarrhoea depends on the answers to four questions and the examination of the patient. First, tell me why each question is useful.

The first question is: **How many times have you passed faeces this morning?**

Student: *If a patient passes loose or watery faeces three times or more in a day, he has diarrhoea. If a patient has passed very watery faeces six times or more today, he may have cholera.*

Trainer: Excellent.

The second question is: **Do you have a fever?**

Student: *The patient may need treatment for the problem which causes the fever. Malaria, pneumonia, tonsillitis, measles and otitis media cause a fever and sometimes cause diarrhoea.*

Trainer: Good.

The third question is: **Is there any blood in your faeces?**

Student: *If there is blood in the diarrhoea, the patient usually has dysentery.*

Trainer: Correct.

The fourth question is: **For how long have you had diarrhoea?**

Student: *If the patient has had diarrhoea for 2 weeks, he has persistent diarrhoea.*

Trainer: Excellent. Then, examine the patient. Next, make sure that he does not have a general danger sign.
  • If the patient has a general danger sign, treat this first.
  • If the patient has blood in his faeces or pain in his abdomen, examine his abdomen. If there is no guarding or rebound tenderness, the patient does not have an abdominal problem. Treat him for dysentery.
How can we tell if a patient is dehydrated?

Student: *If a patient is dehydrated, his mouth is dry. If we pinch a fold of the patient's skin and let go, the skin goes back slowly. If the patient is very dehydrated, the skin takes more than 2 seconds to become flat again.*

Trainer: Good. Children with severe malnutrition also have very loose skin on the abdomen. Pinch a fold of skin over a bone. If you think a patient may be dehydrated or have severe malnutrition, ask what colour his urine is. If the patient is dehydrated, the urine will be dark yellow and he will have passed urine only one time or no times this morning.

Treatment

Trainer: Patients with diarrhoea need treatment to prevent or to treat dehydration and to prevent malnutrition. Patients often get malnutrition after they have had diarrhoea.

Immediate treatment after examination

Trainer: Give a patient with dehydration oral rehydration solution. Give 20 ml of the solution for each kilogram of body weight every hour. Give the solution in small amounts.
Can you tell me for how long we should treat patients?

Student: *Treat patients with severe dehydration for 6 hours using a nasogastric tube. Treat patients with some dehydration for 4 hours using a cup and spoon.*

Trainer: Very good. For example: A 10-kg child will need 200 ml of the solution in each hour. If the child has some dehydration, give a total of 800 ml in 4 hours. If the child has severe dehydration, give a total of 1200 ml in 6 hours.
Treat patients with a *general danger sign* for a very severe febrile disease. Also give a patient who has a general danger sign and diarrhoea 5 ml of oral rehydration solution every minute on the way to the hospital. Use a cup and spoon or a nasogastric tube with a syringe.
If a patient has had diarrhoea six times or more this morning, he may have *cholera*.
- Give oral rehydration solution for 4 to 6 hours. If the patient is no better, send them to a cholera centre.
- Give the first-line antibiotic for cholera 4 to 6 hours after starting treatment with oral rehydration solution. Give antibiotics for 3 days.

If the patient has bloody diarrhoea, but no abdominal problem, he usually has *dysentery:*
- If the patient is a child, treat with co-trimoxazole.
- If the patient is an adult, he does not need medicine. However, if he is no better 5 days after the dysentery started, treat him with co-trimoxazole.
- Treat all patients with malnutrition and dysentery with co-trimoxazole.

POSTER 4: **Co-trimoxazole treatment for dysentery**
(Prepared poster) Copy Table 1 onto Poster 4.

TABLE 1 Co-trimoxazole treatment for dysentery

Age	Dose of co-trimoxazole
Up to 6 months	¼ tablet or 2.5 ml liquid two times a day for 5 days
7 months to 5 years	½ tablet or 5 ml liquid two times a day for 5 days
6 years to 12 years	1 tablet two times a day for 5 days
More than 12 years	2 tablets two times a day for 5 days

Note: 1 tablet = 480 mg = 10 ml liquid

Continue with the demonstration.

Student: *Can I treat all patients with diarrhoea with antibiotics?*

Trainer: No. Only use antibiotics to treat diarrhoea if the patient has dysentery or cholera.

Student: *How should we treat a patient with **persistent diarrhoea?***

Trainer: If the patient is not dehydrated, teach him about home treatment and ask him to go to the hospital this week. If a patient with persistent diarrhoea is dehydrated, treat the dehydration first, then send him to hospital immediately.

Treatment after 4–6 hours

Student: *What do you do after giving the patient oral rehydration solution for 4 or 6 hours?*

Trainer: After treatment, pinch the skin again:
- If the patient still has severe dehydration, send him to hospital for intravenous fluids. Give 5 ml of oral rehydration solution each minute on the way to hospital.
- If the patient still has some dehydration, continue to give oral rehydration solution for another 4 hours.

Student: *How do we treat patients after 4 or 6 hours of treatment who do not have dehydration any more?*

Trainer: We give these patients oral rehydration salts to make up a solution at home. Teach the patient or the patient's mother about home treatment of diarrhoea.

Home treatment

Ask the students how to treat diarrhoea at home. Look for the following answers.

Answer   Give the patient as much extra fluid as he will drink. Tell the mother that if the child vomits, this is usually only one-quarter of the fluid that he has drunk, so that most of the extra fluid is still inside him. If the child is breastfeeding, breastfeed him frequently and for longer than usual at each feed. Give clean water between breastfeeds. The patient's urine should become clear instead of dark and yellow.

Answer   Feed the patient five times a day or more. Continue doing this until the patient is well again and for one extra week after he gets well. This is especially important to prevent malnutrition if the patient is a young child.

Answer   Tell the patient to return to the health centre if the patient:
- cannot drink or breastfeed
- becomes more ill
- develops a fever
- has blood in his faeces.

Continue the demonstration tutorial.

POSTER 5:
(Prepared poster)

Extra fluid for diarrhoea
Copy Table 2 onto Poster 5.

TABLE 2   Extra fluid for diarrhoea

Age	Amount of extra fluid to give each time a patient passes loose faeces
Up to 2 years	100 ml (½ cup)
2 years to 9 years	200 ml (1 cup)
10 years and more	400 ml (2 cups)

Trainer: Teach mothers that children with diarrhoea need more fluid than they normally drink each day. Give extra fluid each time the patient passes loose faeces. Show the mother how much extra fluid to give. What extra fluid should she give if the patient was dehydrated when he arrived at the health centre?

Student: *At first we give oral rehydration solution as extra fluid between feeds.*

Trainer: Excellent. Each standard packet of oral rehydration salts will make 1 litre (1000 ml) of solution. Give two standard packets of oral rehydration salts to children less than 10 years old. Give four standard packets of oral rehydration salts to patients aged 10 or more. Show the mother how to make up the solution. Tell her that the solution or other extra fluids may make diarrhoea worse, but these fluids will prevent dehydration.

Use the instructions in Appendix 11 to teach students how to put in a nasogastric tube. Give the students a copy of Appendix 12.

Refreshment break.

Demonstration

What to teach village leaders
For this demonstration, the volunteer student will teach the class.

POSTER 6:
(Student answer poster)

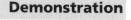
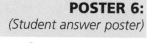
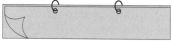

How to prevent diarrhoea
Divide Poster 6 into four areas and write the four headings: '1. How to feed children', '2. Food hygiene', '3. Pit latrines' and '4. Treatment'. The volunteer student will use Poster 6 during this demonstration.

Tell your students:

Imagine you are going to talk to the leaders in your village about preventing diarrhoea. Village leaders are important people. It may be difficult to tell them what to do. Let the village leaders tell you how to prevent people getting ill with diarrhoea.

Now ask the volunteer student to teach the class. She will play the role of the teacher. The other students will play village leaders.

The student teacher says to the village leaders:

Many of us know some of the ways to prevent our children from getting ill or dying with diarrhoea. It is important that we all know *all* the ways to prevent diarrhoea. I would like you to tell me your ideas. Think about your ideas in each of these four areas. I will write your ideas on Poster 6 under the four areas as you call them out.

Ask the student teacher to put up Poster 6.

The student teacher should encourage the village leaders to say the correct answers below. She should also summarise any other useful things that the village leaders say under the correct areas on Poster 6.

Area 1: **How to feed children**
1. **Breastfeed** children **until** they reach **2 years of age**.
2. **Never use a bottle** to feed children. Bottles are very difficult to clean. The bacteria in bottles cause diarrhoea. **Use a cup and a spoon** to give fluids.
3. Feed children **less than 5 months** with **breastmilk only**. After 5 months of age, give children other soft foods in addition to breastmilk. **After 9 months of age** give a **mixed diet** at least **four times a day** in addition to breastmilk.

Area 2: **Food hygiene**
1. Drinking water should be from a **protected water source**. Tap water is normally safe. Water from a well is normally safe if the well has been built correctly. Boil water from any other source for 20 minutes to make it safe to drink.
2. **Wash fruit and vegetables** before eating.
3. **Wash** your **hands** before preparing or eating food.
4. Cover food, faeces and rubbish to keep flies away.

Area 3: **Pit latrines**
1. Go to the toilet or put **all faeces in** a **latrine**. If there is no latrine, use a small hole away from the house. Cover faeces with some soil every day.
2. **Wash** your **hands** after passing faeces. Wash young children after they have passed faeces.
3. If a **child** passes **faeces** near the house put the faeces **in** the **latrine** or hole.

Area 4: **Treatment for diarrhoea**
1. Drink plenty of fluids. Any type of fluid (except alcohol) will help. Sugar and salt solution or coconut water with a pinch of salt are better than normal drinks. Give **as much fluid as** the person **will take** between feeds.
2. **Feed at least five times a day.**
3. **Bring** the patient **to the health centre if**:
   • he is **not able to drink** or breastfeed
   • he becomes **more unwell**
   • he develops a **fever**
   • there is **blood in his faeces**.

Ask students to copy Poster 6 when it is finished.

Polio

Good food hygiene and using pit latrines will also prevent polio.

If polio is a problem in your area, teach Appendix 13 'Polio'.

SECTION 3: When to refer patients to hospital

You should send a patient to hospital if:
1. She has a general danger sign.
2. After 4–6 hours of treatment, the skin still takes more than 2 seconds to become flat again.
3. She has passed very watery faeces six times or more this morning. (Send to a cholera treatment centre.)
4. She has had diarrhoea for more than 2 weeks.
5. She has peritonitis. (Send to a hospital that can do operations.)

SECTION 4: Practical

Tell the students that we will do three role plays to help them diagnose and treat patients with diarrhoea. Divide the class into six groups of at least three students. Each group does each of the three role plays. In each role play, one student will play the doctor, one student will play the patient or the patient's mother, and a third student will be the observer.

Tell your students:

• Give the patient (or the patient's mother) a piece of paper.

This piece of paper tells the patient what symptoms he has. If the doctor asks the correct questions, the patient will tell the doctor about his symptoms.

• Give the doctor a piece of paper.

This piece of paper tells the doctor what she will find when she examines the patient. The doctor's job is to ask the four important questions for diarrhoea. The doctor must make sure that the patient does not have a general danger sign. The doctor decides what treatment to give the patient.

• Give the observer a piece of paper.

This piece of paper tells the observer: (1) the diagnosis, (2) the treatment, (3) advice for the patient, and (4) whether the patient should be sent to hospital. After each role play, the observer should tell the group what the doctor did correctly and what he could have done better.

Role plays

- Tell the groups that they have 40 minutes to do all three role plays. Different students should play each role in each role play.
- Give each group the three role plays and help the students to use Appendix 10. Below is the information for the role plays.

ROLE PLAY 1:

You are the **mother** of the patient, a 6-month-old child. The child has a fever and he has had diarrhoea for 2 days. He passed faeces two times this morning. He does not have blood in his faeces. He vomited one time today. He has not had a convulsion. He passed clear urine two times this morning.

You are the **doctor**. You find that the patient's mouth is not dry. A pinch of skin over his hip bone goes back quickly. The child is breastfeeding. His growth chart shows that he weighs 6½ kg. The growth line is flat but it went up last month.

You are the **observer**. The child has gastroenteritis and possible malaria. Give the child the first-line treatment for malaria. Teach the mother home treatment for diarrhoea.

ROLE PLAY 2:

You are the **mother** of a patient, an 18-month-old child. The child does not have a fever. He has had diarrhoea for 4 days. He has passed very watery faeces four times this morning. He does not have blood in his faeces. He has vomited one time today. He has not passed urine this morning. He breastfeeds slowly.

You are the **doctor**. You find that the patient's mouth is dry. A pinch of skin over his hip bone takes more than 2 seconds to go flat. He is not anaemic and has no fever. His growth chart shows that he now weighs 8½ kg and he weighed 9 kg one month ago.

You are the **observer**. The child has gastroenteritis and severe dehydration. Put in a nasogastric tube. Give oral rehydration solution in small amounts. Give 170 ml (20 ml × 8.5 kg) of this solution every hour for 6 hours. This is a total of 1020 ml (170 × 6). Next, pinch his skin again. If the skin goes back quickly, give home treatment if the child is able to drink. If the skin still takes less than 2 seconds to become flat again, continue to give oral rehydration solution in small amounts. Give him 170 ml of solution every hour for 4 hours. This is a total of 680 ml (170 × 4).

ROLE PLAY 3:

You are the **mother** of a 5-year-old child. The child has a fever. He has had diarrhoea for 2 days. He passed loose faeces three times this morning. He does not have blood in his faeces. He has vomited four times today. He is not able to breastfeed. He has not had a convulsion.

You are the **doctor**. You find that the patient's mouth is dry. A pinch of skin over his hip bone takes less than 2 seconds to go flat. The child has no interest in anything. He is not anaemic. His growth chart shows that he weighs 13 kg.

You are the **observer**. The child has a general danger sign and a very severe febrile disease. Clear his mouth. Lay him on his side. Treat fever with tepid sponging. Give him an intramuscular injection of quinine or chloroquine. Give him an intramuscular injection of chloramphenicol, benzylpenicillin or procaine penicillin fortified. On the way to the hospital, give oral rehydration solution, 5 ml each minute through a nasogastric tube.

SECTION 5: Answers to the quiz

Ask the students to call out the answers to each question in the quiz.

1. When should you use antibiotics to treat patients who have diarrhoea?
   Treat all children with dysentery with co-trimoxazole.
   Treat all patients who have both malnutrition and dysentery with co-trimoxazole.
   Treat very ill adults with co-trimoxazole if they have dysentery.
   Treat adults who are no better 5 days after the dysentery started with co-trimoxazole.
   Antibiotics are also used to treat cholera.

2. What are the causes of diarrhoea?
   - **Gastroenteritis**. Gastroenteritis is caused by bad hygiene. Good hygiene means:
     - wash hands before preparing or eating food
     - use a pit latrine when passing faeces
     - drink water from a protected water source
     - breastfeed, never bottle-feed children
     - wash fruit and vegetables
   - **Food poisoning**
   - **Malnutrition**
   - **Any illness which causes a fever**
     - malaria
     - tonsillitis
     - measles
     - otitis media
   - **Severe illnesses that may cause peritonitis**
     - appendicitis
     - intussusception

3. How can you tell if a patient is dehydrated?
   The patient's mouth is dry.
   Pinch a fold of his skin, over a bone, and let it go. The skin goes back slowly.

4. When should patients with diarrhoea be sent to hospital?
   Patients with a general danger sign.
   If, after treating a patient for 4–6 hours, the skin takes more than 2 seconds to become flat again.
   The patient has passed very watery faeces six times or more this morning. (Send to a cholera treatment centre.)
   If a patient has had diarrhoea for more than 2 weeks.
   If a patient has peritonitis. (Send to a hospital that can do operations.)

Women's health problems

BEFORE THE LESSON

■ There are two posters in this lesson. (See p. 4 for information on how to use the posters.)

■ Prepared posters: 1, 2

■ Make a copy for each student of Appendixes 14 and 15.

■ There are nine demonstrations in section 2. Ask nine students to help you. Prepare two copies of each role play. Give one copy to a student. The other copy is for you (or use this book). Practise before the lesson.

■ Decide if you need to teach students how to measure haemoglobin (this is not covered in this manual).

■ Prepare two examples of obstetric problems which you will present to students in section 3. Use Appendix 15.

■ Prepare three large signs for the practical in section 4. Prepare one page of paper with a symptom written on it for each student. You need sticky tape.

SECTION 1: Quiz

POSTER 1:
(Prepared poster)

Quiz
Ask the students to answer the questions on their own. Do not give the answers until the end of the lesson.

> 1. Which medicines are safe to give to a pregnant woman?
>
> 2. Which medicines are not safe to give to a woman who is breastfeeding?
>
> 3. How do you treat a pregnant woman who is having a convulsion?
>
> 4. How do you treat anaemia in the last month of pregnancy?

SECTION 2: Diagnosis and management

Discussion

In some countries, it may be difficult for a male health worker to treat a woman patient who has gynaecological problems (problems with her private parts). Divide the students into three groups. Ask the groups to discuss how this difficulty can be solved in your country. Next, ask each group to present their ideas.

Gynaecology problems

Women who are not pregnant may have problems with their private parts. These are called gynaecology problems. Pain in the lower abdomen or an unusual discharge from the private parts are usually gynaecology problems. Take a history. You then need to ask women with these problems five questions (see Poster 2).

POSTER 2:
(Prepared poster)

Questions for women with gynaecology problems

1. For how many days do you bleed each month? Does blood make your pad or cloth very wet in less than one hour?
2. Do you have bad pain every month when your period comes?
3. Is it painful when you have sexual intercourse? Do you pass blood after sexual intercourse when you do not have a period?
4. Do you have an unusual or smelly discharge from your private parts?
5. Was your last normal period more than 6 weeks ago?

Tell the students that we will now discuss the answers to these questions and what treatment to give. Give each student a copy of Appendix 14.

1. If a woman bleeds for more than 8 days every month or if a pad or cloth becomes very wet in less than one hour, she has **heavy periods**. Heavy periods may cause anaemia. Check for anaemia and treat if present.
   Treatment:
   - If the woman plans to get pregnant, give her ibuprofen 400 mg three times a day (after food) *only* on the days that she has pain or bleeding.
   - If the woman does not plan to get pregnant, send her to the Maternal and Child Health or family planning clinic. The clinic may give her the combined oral contraceptive pill. Taking the pill will stop her from bleeding heavily. For most women it is safe to take the combined oral contraceptive pill for many years. Women should not take the pill if they are older than 45 years or if they smoke and are older than 40 years.

2. **Pain every month** that stops her from working.
   Treatment:
   - If the woman plans to get pregnant, give her ibuprofen 400 mg three times a day (after food) *only* on the days that she has pain or bleeding.

- If the woman does not plan to get pregnant, send her to the Maternal and Child Health or family planning clinic. The combined oral contraceptive pill will reduce period pain.

3. **Pain or blood during sexual intercourse**.
   Treatment:
   - If the woman is less than 45 years old, she may have a sexually transmitted disease. Send her and her partner to the sexually transmitted disease clinic.
   - If she is more than 45 years old, send her to the gynaecology clinic.

4. Unusual or smelly **discharge from** her **private parts.**
   Treatment:
   - If the woman is less than 45 years old, she may have a sexually transmitted disease. Send her and her partner to the sexually transmitted disease clinic.
   - If she is more than 45 years old, send her to the gynaecology clinic.

5. **Last** normal **period** was **more than 6 weeks ago.**
   Treatment:
   - If she is less than 45 years old and has pain in her lower abdomen, she may have an ectopic pregnancy (see later in this lesson). Send her to a hospital where operations are done.
   - If she is more than 45 years old, her last period was more than 1 year ago and she is now bleeding again, send her to the gynaecology clinic.

Obstetric problems

Obstetrics is to do with the problems of the private parts of women who are pregnant.

Demonstrations

Give each student a copy of Appendix 15. You will do the following nine demonstrations with different students. The demonstrations show different obstetric problems.

Appendix 15 summarises the main diagnostic and treatment points of these demonstrations. Students will learn how to use Appendix 15 in section 3 of the lesson.

DEMONSTRATION 1: *Vomiting in early pregnancy*

Student: *An 18-year-old woman comes to see you. Her last period was 6 weeks ago. She has vomited two times each day for the past 2 weeks. She does not have any pain when she passes urine. She passes urine more often than usual. Can you help her?*

Trainer: This woman may be pregnant. Vomiting in early pregnancy is a very common problem. If a woman vomits severely in pregnancy we must look for a urinary tract infection. Send her to have her urine examined. If she has a urinary tract infection, give her amoxicillin 250 mg three times a day for 5 days.

Student: *Are there any other problems that cause severe vomiting in pregnancy?*

Trainer: Twin pregnancy may cause severe vomiting.

Student: *If the woman does not have a urinary tract infection, what treatment can we give her?*

Trainer: Send her to hospital if she is vomiting severely. Advise her to eat small amounts of food and drink every hour. Tell the woman that this problem will usually disappear before 14 weeks after the start of her last period. Do not give her any medicine. Medicines to stop vomiting can damage the unborn baby.

DEMONSTRATION 2:   *Ectopic pregnancy*

Student: *A 19-year-old woman has had dizziness and severe pain in her lower abdomen for 6 hours. What questions would you ask her? How would you treat her?*

Trainer: Was your last normal period more than 6 weeks ago? If she says yes, she may be pregnant. If she has severe pain in her lower abdomen, she may have an ectopic pregnancy. Send her immediately to a hospital that can do operations. Give her oral rehydration solution, one teaspoonful every minute.

An ectopic pregnancy means that the unborn baby is not inside the uterus. This is very dangerous because ectopic pregnancy may cause bleeding inside the abdomen, peritonitis and shock. A woman with shock may feel dizzy, anxious and sweaty. She may lose consciousness. An operation may save the woman's life.

DEMONSTRATION 3:   *Antepartum haemorrhage (APH)*

Student: *A woman who is 7 months pregnant has passed a small amount of blood from her private parts. She does not have pain in her abdomen. She does not have a fever. What would you do for her?*

Trainer: This woman has had an antepartum (before birth) haemorrhage. Send her to hospital immediately.

Student: *What would you do if the woman started to bleed heavily?*

Trainer: Give her oral rehydration solution to drink. She should drink one teaspoonful every minute on her way to hospital.

Student: *Another woman who is less than 6 months pregnant passes blood from her private parts. What would you do?*

Trainer: This is either a threatened abortion or an abortion. An abortion is when the unborn baby dies.
- If the woman has a fever, give her an intramuscular injection of 2 million IU of benzylpenicillin. Next, send her to hospital.
- If the woman passes more than a small amount of blood, send her to hospital.
- If the woman does not have a fever and only passes a small amount of blood, tell her to rest at home. She should not do any heavy work or have sexual intercourse for 2 weeks.

DEMONSTRATION 4: *Anaemia in pregnancy*

(You may want to teach students how to measure haemoglobin. This is not covered in this manual.)

Student: *A woman who is in the last month of her pregnancy feels weak and tired. She is pale. How would you treat her?*

Trainer: Measure the woman's haemoglobin (Hb) in the health centre or hospital. Examine the woman's faeces for hookworm eggs.
1. If her haemoglobin is less than 7 g/dl give her the first-line malaria treatment in malaria areas. Next, send her to hospital for a blood transfusion.
2. If her haemoglobin is between 7 g/dl and 10 g/dl:
   - Give her the first-line malaria treatment if there is malaria in your area and she has a fever.
   - Give her mebendazole if there are many hookworm eggs in the faeces. Do not give mebendazole in the first 3 months of pregnancy.
   - Give her ferrous sulphate 200 mg (with or without folic acid 0.25 mg) three times a day for at least 3 months.

Student: *Is it possible to stop pregnant women from becoming anaemic?*

Trainer: Yes. Teach women to eat a mixed diet with foods that contain iron, folic acid and vitamin C. Advise women to wear shoes. Give pregnant women 200 mg ferrous sulphate and 0.4 mg of folic acid (or one tablet of ferrous sulphate 200 mg with folic acid 0.25 mg) every day for the whole of the pregnancy in areas where iron deficiency is common.

DEMONSTRATION 5: *Pre-eclampsia and eclampsia*

Student: *A woman who is 8 months pregnant has a headache. She does not have a fever. Her diastolic blood pressure is 100 mmHg. She may have pre-eclampsia. What should you do for her?*

Trainer: Send any pregnant woman with a diastolic blood pressure of 100 mmHg or more to hospital immediately. If a pregnant woman's blood pressure goes very high she may have a convulsion. This is called eclampsia. Eclampsia may kill her and her unborn baby.

Student: *What causes pre-eclampsia and eclampsia?*

Trainer: The cause is not known. Pre-eclampsia and eclampsia damage the kidneys, the blood vessels and the brain. The kidney damage causes women to pass protein in their urine. The blood vessel damage causes women to have high blood pressure. The brain damage causes convulsions and death.

Student: *How can we stop eclampsia from killing women?*

Trainer: The Maternal and Child Health worker should measure a pregnant woman's blood pressure every second week in the last 3 months of pregnancy.

- If the woman's diastolic blood pressure is 90 mmHg or more, examine the blood pressure again after one week.
- If the blood pressure is 95 mmHg or more, send the woman to hospital this week.
- If the blood pressure is 100 mmHg or more, send the woman to hospital today.

Student: *What should we do if a pregnant woman has a convulsion?*

Trainer:
- Give her 10 mg diazepam rectally.
- Next, put her onto her side so that if she vomits she will not breathe in the vomit.
- Give her magnesium sulphate 5 g intramuscularly into each leg.
- Send her to a hospital where operations are done.
- If she is still having a convulsion after 5 minutes, give her 10 mg diazepam rectally again.
- Give a further 5 g of magnesium sulphate after 4 hours, 2.5 g into each leg.

DEMONSTRATION 6: *Prolapsed cord*

Student: *A woman who is in the last month of her pregnancy tells you that a large amount of water passed from her private parts today. The baby's umbilical cord is hanging out of the woman's private parts. What will you do?*

Trainer: What you do depends on whether the cord has a pulse:
- If the umbilical cord does not have a pulse, the baby is already dead. The woman may be able to give birth to the dead baby at home. If the baby has not been born after 12 hours send her to hospital.
- If the umbilical cord has a pulse and the cervix is fully open (10 cm wide), allow the baby to be born immediately.
- If the umbilical cord has a pulse and the cervix is not fully open, ask the woman to kneel down and to bend forward. Her bottom should be higher than her head. Gently put the umbilical cord back into the woman's private parts. Gently push the baby away from the cord. Next, send the woman to a hospital where operations are done immediately. The woman will have to be carried very carefully.

Refreshment break

DEMONSTRATION 7: *Ruptured uterus*

Student: *A 30-year-old woman who has already had seven children has been in labour for 24 hours. She had severe, constant pain in her abdomen. The woman lost consciousness 10 minutes ago.*

Trainer: The woman's uterus may have ruptured. You may be able to feel parts of the baby's body very easily in the woman's abdomen. Her pulse will be fast and weak. Her blood pressure will be low. The woman may pass blood from her private parts.

Student: *What would you do for her?*

Trainer: Send her immediately to a hospital where operations are done. If possible, give her intravenous fluids. (If the woman is conscious, give her oral rehydration solution to drink, 5 ml every minute.)

She must go to hospital urgently. There is a high chance that she will die.

Student: *How can we prevent the uterus from rupturing?*

Trainer: Send the patient to a hospital where operations are done:
- If a woman's labour pain has been happening regularly for more than one day and one night.
- If a woman has been pushing for more than 2 hours with no progress.

DEMONSTRATION 8: *Postpartum haemorrhage (PPH)*

Student: *A 35-year-old woman gave birth to her seventh child half an hour ago. The woman has a large amount of blood coming from her private parts. She feels dizzy.*

Trainer: This is called postpartum haemorrhage.
- Tell the woman to pass urine immediately where she is.
- Tell her to breastfeed the child immediately. If the child is dead, ask her to squeeze her nipples between her fingers.
- Give her an injection of 0.5 mg ergometrine into a vein or intramuscularly.
- Give her oral rehydration solution to drink, 5 ml every minute.
- If the placenta does not come out, send the woman to a hospital where operations are done.

Show the students what you mean in the next point, pretending to put your hands on the woman's uterus. Ask them also to copy your actions.

- If the bleeding has not stopped and the placenta has come out, feel the uterus in the abdomen. If the uterus is soft, put your right hand into her private parts and squeeze the uterus with your left hand. If the uterus stays soft, continue to squeeze until the woman sees a women's doctor. If the uterus is hard, put a clean cloth into her vagina to stop blood from coming out. Take the woman immediately to a hospital where operations are done.

Student: *If a woman starts to bleed heavily from her private parts more than 24 hours after the baby was born, what would you do?*

Trainer: Send the woman to hospital.

DEMONSTRATION 9: *Medicines for pregnant women and women who are breastfeeding*

Student: *A 25-year-old woman who is 2½ months pregnant was treated with the first-line malaria treatment less than 2 weeks ago. She has a fever. A blood test shows that she has malaria. What treatment can you safely use?*

Trainer: Quinine. Chloroquine is also safe to use in pregnancy. If Fansidar is the first-line malaria treatment, only give Fansidar if you do not have quinine.

Student: *What other medicines are safe to use for pregnant women?*

Trainer:	Paracetamol, aluminium hydroxide, phenoxymethylpenicillin, benzylpenicillin, amoxicillin, ampicillin, ferrous sulphate, folic acid, oral rehydration salts solution, and most medicines which are put on the skin. Fansidar is safe *after* the first 3 months of pregnancy.
Student:	*What medicines are not safe to give to women who are breastfeeding or pregnant?*
Trainer:	Chloramphenicol and the combined oral contraceptive pill.

SECTION 3:   When to refer patients to hospital

Teach student how to use Appendix 15. Give the students two examples of obstetric problems and show them how to use the appendix for diagnosis and treatment.

SECTION 4:   Practical

This activity will help you to learn the symptoms of sexually transmitted diseases and urinary tract infections.

Give each student a piece of paper with a number and one of the following nine symptoms written on it. For example, if you have 27 students, you need three pieces of paper with each symptom.

1. Unusual discharge from the private parts.
2. Pain when having sexual intercourse.
3. Ulcers near the private parts.
4. Pain on passing urine.
5. Passes urine more often than usual.
6. Pain in the lower abdomen.
7. Fever.
8. The woman's partner has pain when he passes urine.
9. The woman's partner has a discharge from his private parts.

Activity

Ask each student to stick the paper on their chest. Put a large sign 'Sexually transmitted disease' on one wall. On the opposite wall, put a sign 'Urinary tract infection'. On a wall between these two walls, put a sign 'Sexually transmitted disease or Urinary tract infection'.

Explain that the symptom each student has written on the paper on their chest may be caused by either a sexually transmitted disease or a urinary tract infection or by both.

Tell the students:
- If you think that your symptom can *only* be caused by a sexually transmitted disease, stand by that sign.
  Answer   Students with numbers 1, 2, 3, 8 and 9 should stand next to the 'Sexually transmitted disease' sign.
- If you think that your symptom can only be caused by a urinary tract infection, stand by that sign.
  Answer   No students stand next to the 'Urinary tract infection' sign.

- If you think that your symptom can be caused by *either* a sexually transmitted disease or a urinary tract infection, stand by the third sign.
  Answer   Students with numbers 4, 5, 6 and 7 stand next to the 'Sexually transmitted disease or Urinary tract infection' sign.

Treatment:
- If a patient has symptom 1, 2, 3, 8 or 9 (say the symptoms) send her and her partner to the sexually transmitted disease clinic.
- If a patient has symptom 4 or 5 (say the symptoms), send her to have her urine examined. She may have a urinary tract infection.

SECTION 5:   Answers to the quiz

Ask the students to call out the answers to each question in the quiz.

1. Which medicines are safe to give to a pregnant woman?
   Quinine, chloroquine, paracetamol, aluminium hydroxide, phenoxymethylpenicillin, benzylpenicillin, amoxicillin, ampicillin, ferrous sulphate, folic acid, oral rehydration salts solution and most medicines which are put on the skin. Fansidar is safe after the first 3 months of pregnancy.

2. Which medicines are not safe to give to women who are breastfeeding?
   Chloramphenicol and the combined oral contraceptive pill.

3. How do you treat a pregnant woman who is having a convulsion?
   - **Give her diazepam 10 mg rectally.**
   - **Next, put her onto her side.**
   - **Give her magnesium sulphate 5 g intramuscularly *into each* leg.**
   - **Send her to a hospital where operations are done.**
   - **If she is still having a convulsion after 5 minutes, give her diazepam 10 mg rectally again.**
   - **Give a further 5 g of magnesium sulphate after 4 hours, 2.5 g into each leg.**

4. How do you treat anaemia in the last month of pregnancy?
   Measure the woman's haemoglobin. Check to see if she has a fever. Look for hookworm in the woman's faeces.
   - **If her haemoglobin is less than 7 g/dl give her the first line malaria treatment if there is malaria in the area, and send her to hospital for a blood transfusion.**
   - **If there is malaria in the area, give a patient with fever the first-line malaria treatment.**
   - **If there are a large number of hookworm eggs in the faeces, give mebendazole**
   - **If her haemoglobin is 7 g/dl or more and below 10 g/dl give her ferrous sulphate 200 mg three times a day for at least 3 months.**

Lesson 8 Abdominal problems

BEFORE THE LESSON

- There are nine posters in this lesson. (See p. 4 for information on how to use the posters.)
  Prepared posters: 1, 4, 6, 9
  Student answer posters: 2, 3, 7, 8
  Summary poster: 5

- For Sections 2 and 3, you need a long sock and two balls of different sizes. Cut the end off the sock.

- You need a table or a bed at the front of the class for the demonstration 'How to examine the abdomen' in Section 2. Ask a male student to help you with the demonstration and practise before the lesson.

- Ask a male student to volunteer to allow you to draw the numbers of a clock on his abdomen.

- Prepare a copy of Pictures 15 and 16 for each student.

- Prepare a blank copy of Table 3, 'Features of abdominal problems', for each student. Copy the headings only and leave the boxes empty.

- If diabetes is a problem in your area, make a copy of Appendix 16 for each student.

- If your students can do urine microscopy in their health centres, make a copy of Appendix 17 for each student.

- Make a copy of Appendix 18 for each student.

- Prepare two examples of abdominal problems which you will present in section 3. Use Appendix 18.

- For Section 4, you need one copy of the questions for each group of five students.

SECTION 1: Quiz

POSTER 1:
(Prepared poster)

Quiz

Ask the students to answer the questions on their own. Do not give the answers until the end of the lesson.

1. Name eight causes of peritonitis.
2. A woman has abdominal pain. What questions should you ask her?

SECTION 2: Diagnosis and management

Abdominal pain

Almost all abdominal problems cause abdominal pain. To diagnose the cause of abdominal pain, we need to know what type of pain each abdominal problem causes, and where each abdominal problem causes pain.

There are two main types of abdominal pain:

- intermittent abdominal pain
- constant abdominal pain.

Intermittent abdominal pain

Abdominal pain is intermittent if it becomes bad for a short time (several seconds or a minute) and then gets better. The pain increases and decreases. Intermittent pain can continue for several hours or a few days. Patients with intermittent abdominal pain find it difficult to sit still. Intermittent pain may be caused by irritation or blockage of the bowel inside the abdomen. It may also be caused by problems in the ureters.

You now use the sock and the two balls to demonstrate how a blocked bowel can cause intermittent pain. Put the small ball inside the sock. Tell the students that this long sock is like the bowel. The bowel pushes food or faeces along. Normally food or faeces is soft and small and the bowel can easily push it. This small ball is like a small piece of food or faeces inside the bowel. Press on the ball and show the students how easy it is to push the ball from one end of the sock to the other. Explain that in the same way, it is easy for the bowel to push soft, small food or faeces. This does not cause pain.
Put the large ball inside the sock. Tell the students that it is difficult for the bowel to push through faeces that are hard and large. The large ball is like a large piece of faeces inside the bowel. Press on the ball and show the students that it is very difficult to push the ball from one end of the sock to the other. The bowel tries to push intermittently and this causes intermittent pain.

Next, you will teach the students where different abdominal problems cause pain. Ask the student who volunteered to have the numbers of the clock drawn on his abdomen to take off his shirt and to show the class where you have put each number (Picture 14).

POSTER 2:
(Student answer poster)

Intermittent abdominal pain
Write the *headings and the left column only* of Table 1 (p. 106) on Poster 2. Ask the students where each abdominal problem causes pain.

Constant abdominal pain

Other abdominal problems usually cause constant abdominal pain. Constant pain is pain that does not go away. Patients with constant abdominal pain usually stay still.

POSTER 3:
(Student answer poster)

Constant abdominal pain
Write the *headings and the left column only* of Table 2 (p. 107) on Poster 3. Ask the students where each abdominal problem causes pain.
Next, give each student a copy of Pictures 15 and 16.

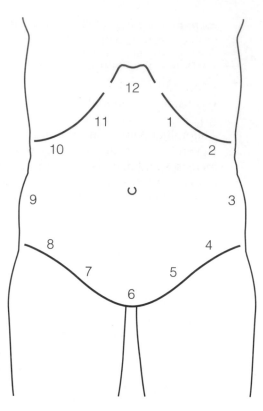

PICTURE 14 *Areas of the abdomen*

TABLE 1 Intermittent abdominal pain

Abdominal problems that cause intermittent pain	Where the problem causes pain
Labour (the pains that push the baby out when a baby is born)	6 and in the lower back
Early appendicitis	In the centre
Intussusception	In the centre
Volvulus	In the centre or 6
Gastroenteritis and food poisoning	12, in the centre or 6
Constipation	4, 5 or 6
Early incarcerated hernia	In the centre or 6
Kidney stones (stones in a ureter)	3 or 9

TABLE 2   Constant abdominal pain

Abdominal problems that cause constant pain	Where the problem causes pain
Peritonitis	Any area then all of the abdomen
Late appendicitis	7 and 8 then all of the abdomen
Urinary tract infection	6
Kidney infection (pyelonephritis)	3 or 9
Pelvic inflammatory disease (PID)	5, 6 or 7
Ectopic pregnancy	5, 6 or 7 then all of the abdomen
Peptic ulcer or gastritis	12
Late incarcerated hernia	5, 6 or 7 then all of the abdomen
Typhoid	Any area then all of the abdomen
Hepatitis	10 or 11

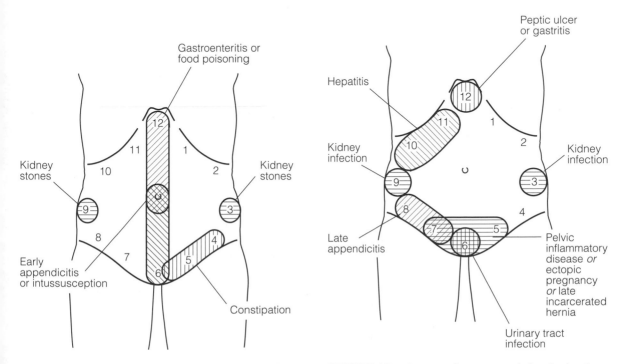

PICTURE 15   *Causes of intermittent abdominal pain*

PICTURE 16   *Causes of constant abdominal pain*

How to take an abdominal history

Questions to ask patients with abdominal pain or with blood in the faeces

1. Do you have any problems when you pass urine?
2. Are your bowels all right?
3. If the patient is a woman, ask: When was your last normal menstrual period? Does your pain come at the same time as your period? Is it painful when you have sexual intercourse?
4. Show me where you feel the pain.
5. What type of pain do you feel? Is the pain constant or intermittent?
6. Is there anyone else at home who has the same symptoms that you have?

How to examine the abdomen

After taking a history, examine the abdomen of all patients who have severe abdominal pain or blood in the faeces.

Demonstration

Tell the students that you will show them how to do an examination. Put a bed or table at the front of the class. Ask the student with clock numbers drawn on his abdomen to walk towards you slowly. Tell him to hold his stomach and bend slightly forward as he walks. Ask him to slowly get onto the bed and lie on his back. Examine the volunteer with your right hand.

How to examine patients with severe abdominal pain

This patient bends forward when he walks, because he has severe abdominal pain. Do the following:

1. Look for **fever** and **anaemia**.
2. Next, ask the patient to look upwards. If the white part of his eye is yellow, the patient has **jaundice**. Only look for jaundice in sunlight.
3. Ask the patient to **lie flat** on his back with his arms by his side.
4. **Remove the clothes** from the **whole abdomen**. Remove clothes from the private parts of a man. (*Do not ask the student volunteer to do this in the class.*)
5. **Look for scars** of previous operations. Look for **swellings**.

(continued)
6. **Ask** the patient **if** he has any **pain** at the moment. Ask him **where** the pain is.
7. **Watch** the patient's **face** when you touch his abdomen. The patient's face will show you if the patient is in pain.
8. **Use** the part of your **hand** that is best at feeling to do the examination. Start to examine the abdomen in the places where there is least pain.

Show the students, using your hand as an example, the area of the hand that is shown in the Picture 17.

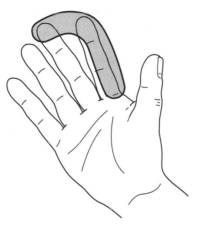

PICTURE 17   *Area of the hand used to examine the abdomen*

POSTER 6:
(Prepared poster)

Four areas of the abdomen
Draw Picture 18 on Poster 6.

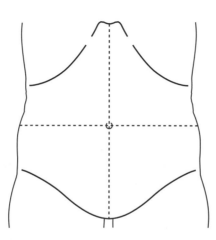

PICTURE 18   *Four areas of the abdomen*

(*continued*)

9. **Examine** each of the four areas of the **abdomen** (Picture 18). First, press lightly into each of the four areas. Next, press more deeply into each of these areas. Look to see if the pain becomes worse when you press. Feel for any unusual swelling.

10. If the pain becomes worse when you press into the abdomen, look for **guarding** and **rebound tenderness**:
    - Press slowly and deeply into the abdomen. If the patient has guarding, the muscles will stop you from examining deeply. Guarding is when the muscles at the front of the abdomen become hard to protect the abdomen from more pain.
    - Press slowly and deeply into the abdomen. Suddenly remove your hand. If the patient has rebound tenderness, the pain will suddenly become worse. Watch the patient's face.

11. Look for a **large spleen**. Start at area 7. Press your hand into the abdomen. Move your hand a little towards area 2. Press the abdomen again. Do this again and again. If the patient has a large spleen, you will feel the hard edge of the spleen before you feel the edge of the ribs.

12. Look for a **large liver**. Start at area 10. Press your hand into the abdomen. Move your hand a little towards area 11. Press the abdomen again. Do this again and again. If the patient has a large liver you will feel the hard edge of the liver before you feel the edge of the ribs. The liver may also be tender if the patient has hepatitis.

13. Look for **painful kidneys**. Put your left hand behind area 3. Place your right hand on area 3. Press your right hand into the abdomen. If the patient has painful kidneys, the pain will increase when you press. Do the same at area 9.

Common and important abdominal problems

Show the students Poster 4 again.

POSTER 7:
(Student answer poster)

Common and important abdominal problems

Draw the *lines and headings only* of Table 3 (pp. 112–113) on Poster 7. Give each of your students one *blank* copy of Table 3. Students should complete their blank Table 3 with the correct answers.

Labour

Labour pains (also called contractions) push the baby out when a woman is giving birth. A woman in labour will often have

intermittent pain in the low back and the lower abdomen
(area 6). Labour starts when the pains become regular. There are
usually a few minutes between each pain.

Ask the students what to write in each space of the labour row of
the table. Fill in the correct answers on Poster 7. Students should
fill in the correct answers in their blank Table 3.

Peritonitis

Peritonitis is caused by damage or irritation to the inside of the
abdomen. The inside of the abdomen is called the peritoneum.
Peritonitis causes severe abdominal pain. Patients with peritonitis
may vomit, but do not usually have diarrhoea. Patients with
peritonitis often die. If a patient has guarding or rebound
tenderness, he usually has peritonitis.
   Peritonitis is caused by:
- any illness which allows the bacteria or the acid in the
  bowel to enter the peritoneum
- any illness which causes a lot of blood to collect in the
  peritoneum.

POSTER 8:
(Student answer poster)

Causes of peritonitis
Ask your students which eight illnesses commonly cause peritonitis.

Answer
Answer
Answer
Answer
Answer
Answer
Answer
Answer

- **appendicitis**
- **perforated peptic ulcer**
- **intussusception**
- **incarcerated hernia**
- **ectopic pregnancy**
- **pelvic inflammatory disease** (a sexually transmitted disease)
- **typhoid**
- **volvulus**

Send all patients who have guarding or rebound tenderness
immediately to a hospital that can operate. An operation may
prevent death.

Appendicitis
Appendicitis is caused by unusual bacteria which damage the
appendix. If the appendix is damaged, bacteria can enter the
peritoneum and cause peritonitis.

Diagnosis: Appendicitis starts with an intermittent pain in the
centre of the abdomen. After a few hours or days, the pain
becomes constant in area 7 or 8 of the abdomen. The patient
will have a slight fever. He will also have guarding and
rebound tenderness, starting in areas 7 and 8. Later he will
have guarding and rebound tenderness in all areas of the
abdomen.

TABLE 3 Common and important abdominal problems

Problem	Question						
				Pain			
	Problems when pass urine?	Bowels all right?	Last period normal?	Where?	Constant or intermittent?	Anyone else?	May cause peritonitis
Labour				6 and the low back	Intermittent		
Appendicitis				Centre then 7 and 8	Intermittent then constant		Yes
Peptic ulcer or gastritis				12	Constant		Yes
Intussusception		No. Blood		Centre	Intermittent then constant		Yes
Incarcerated hernia		No. Less often		Centre or 6 then 5, 6 or 7	Intermittent then constant		Yes
Ectopic pregnancy			No. Last period missed or unusual	5, 6 or 7 then all of the abdomen	Constant		Yes
Pelvic inflammatory disease			Yes. Pain with sex	5, 6 or 7	Constant		Yes
Typhoid		No. Less often usually		If develops peritonitis any area, then all of the abdomen	Constant if has peritonitis	Sometimes	Yes

TABLE 3 Common and important abdominal problems (*continued*)

Problem	Question				Pain			May cause peritonitis
	Problems when pass urine?	Bowels all right?	Last period normal?	Where?	Constant or intermittent?	Anyone else?		
Volvulus		No. Less often		Centre or 6 then all of the abdomen	Intermittent then constant			Yes
Gastroenteritis and food poisoning		No. Diarrhoea		12, centre and 6	Intermittent	Yes, often		
Constipation		No. Pain. Less often		4, 5 or 6	Intermittent			
Urinary tract infection	Yes. Pain. Passes urine often			6	Constant			
Kidney infection (Pyelonephritis)	Yes. Pain. Passes urine often			3 or 9	Constant			
Kidney stones (stones in a ureter)				3 or 9	Intermittent			
Hepatitis				10 or 11	Constant			
Rectal prolapse		No. Something at anus			No pain in abdomen			

Treatment: Send all patients who may have appendicitis immediately to a hospital where operations are done.

Ask the students what to write in each space of the appendicitis row of the table. Fill in the correct answers on Poster 7. Students should fill in the correct answers in their blank Table 3.

Peptic ulcer or gastritis

Peptic ulcers and gastritis are irritations of the inside of the upper parts of the bowel. Peptic ulcers and gastritis develop if the upper bowel is not able to protect itself from the acid in the stomach. Some medicines, especially ibuprofen and aspirin, and smoking can prevent the stomach from protecting itself. A perforated gastric ulcer is caused when the acid makes a deep hole in the wall of the upper bowel. The acid may reach the outside of the bowel and cause peritonitis.

Diagnosis: The patient has constant pain in area 12 of the abdomen. The pain is made better by eating or drinking. Make the diagnosis from the history. You will not usually find anything when you examine the patient.

Treatment:
- Send all patients with peritonitis immediately to a hospital where operations are done.
- Or: If there is no guarding or rebound tenderness, give the patient aluminium hydroxide. Give him 30 tablets. Tell the patient to chew and swallow one tablet every time he gets the pain.
- Or: If pain in area 12 has been present for 2 weeks or more, the patient may need other treatment for a peptic ulcer. Send the patient to hospital.

Tell all patients with a peptic ulcer or gastritis not to use aspirin or ibuprofen. Tell patients not to smoke. Tell patients who have pain in area 12 to eat small meals frequently and to drink milk.
Ask the students what to write in each space of the ulcer and gastritis row of the table. Fill in the correct answers on Poster 7. Students should fill in the correct answers in their blank Table 3.

Intussusception

Show the students what happens to the bowel in intussusception. Cut the end off a long sock before the lesson. The sock represents the bowel. Show that part of the bowel swallows another part of the bowel (Picture 19).

Intussusception is where one part of the bowel swallows another part. This usually happens near the appendix. Intussusception is very dangerous. It can stop blood reaching part of the bowel and, if this happens, that part of the bowel will die. Later, food and faeces will leak out of the bowel, causing peritonitis.

Diagnosis: When you examine the abdomen you may feel a swelling to the right of the centre of the abdomen.

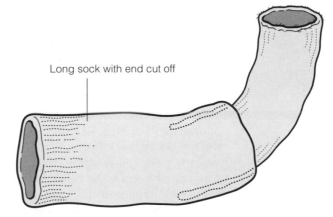

PICTURE 19 *How intussusception happens*

Treatment: Send patients who have a swelling and pain in the abdomen immediately to a hospital where operations are done. Intussusception causes an intermittent pain in the centre of the abdomen. Later, the pain may become constant. The patient may also pass blood with his faeces.

Ask the students what to write in each space of the intussusception row of the table. Fill in the correct answers on Poster 7. Students should fill in the correct answers in their blank Table 3.

Incarcerated hernia

Men often get swellings in the scrotum. These swellings are commonly caused by a hernia, hydrocoele or orchitis. Women can also get hernias.

POSTER 9:
(Prepared poster)

Swellings

Copy pictures 20, 21 and 22 onto Poster 9.

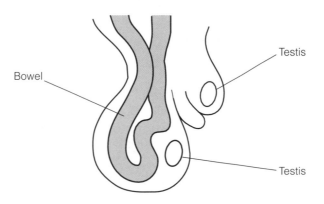

PICTURE 20 *Hernia*

● *Hernia*

A hernia is when part of the bowel comes through a weakness in the bottom of the abdomen into the scrotum or at the fold

115

between the abdomen and the leg. A hernia is usually a painless swelling. The hernia may become incarcerated (trapped) and painful. An incarcerated hernia is a painful swelling which is normally near the private parts.

Diagnosis: Feel at the top of the scrotum or at the fold between the abdomen and the leg. Lay the patient down. Try to push the swelling slowly back into the abdomen. With a hernia, you can normally push the swelling back into the abdomen. With an incarcerated hernia, the bowel does not go back into the abdomen. This is very dangerous because it may stop blood from reaching part of the bowel. This will cause peritonitis.

Treatment:
- If a patient has a painful swelling near the private parts, send him immediately to a hospital where operations are done.
- If a patient has a painless hernia, send him to surgical outpatients at hospital.

Ask the students what to write in each space of the incarcerated hernia row of the table. Fill in the correct answers on Poster 7. Students should fill in the correct answers in their blank Table 3.

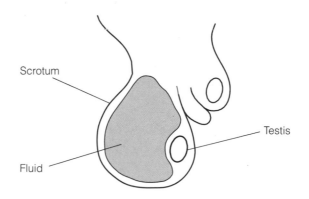

PICTURE 21   *Hydrocoele*

- *Hydrocoele*
A hydrocoele is a bag of fluid in the scrotum. It is usually caused by filarial worms. Filarial worms are transmitted by a mosquito. The worms block lymph vessels and prevent fluid leaving the scrotum.

Diagnosis: Hydrocoeles are not painful. You can feel the top of a hydrocoele at the top of the scrotum. Lay the patient down. Try to push the swelling slowly back into the abdomen. You cannot push a hydrocoele back into the abdomen when the patient is lying down.

Treatment: Send patients with a very large hydrocoele to surgical outpatients at hospital.

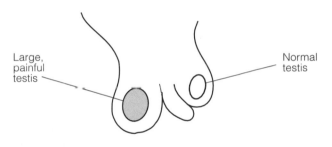

PICTURE 22   *Orchitis*

● *Orchitis*

Orchitis is an infection of one or both testes (testicles).

Diagnosis: The testicle or testicles are large and painful to touch. There may be discharge from the penis and pain when the patient passes urine.

Treatment:

- If a patient with orchitis has pain when he passes urine or a discharge from his penis, send him to the sexually transmitted disease clinic. Ask the patient's partner to go with him.
- Treat all other patients with co-trimoxazole. Give 960 mg (two tablets) two times a day for 5 days.

Ectopic pregnancy

Ectopic pregnancy causes a constant pain in area 5, 6 or 7. If a woman has pain in area 5, 6 or 7, ask about her last period. If her last normal period was more than 6 weeks ago, she may be pregnant and have an ectopic pregnancy (see Lesson 7). Send her immediately to a hospital where operations are done. Give her 5 ml oral rehydration solution every minute.

Ask the students what to write in each space of the ectopic pregnancy row of the table. Fill in the correct answers on Poster 7. Students should fill in the correct answers in their blank Table 3.

Pelvic inflammatory disease (PID)

Pelvic inflammatory disease is a sexually transmitted disease. The uterus and the fallopian tubes are infected. If the infection in the fallopian tubes reaches the peritoneum, the patient may develop peritonitis.

Diagnosis: Pelvic inflammatory disease causes constant pain in area 5, 6 or 7. This pain is worse during sexual intercourse.

Treatment: Send her to the sexually transmitted disease clinic. Ask her partner to go with her.

Ask the students what to write in each space of the pelvic inflammatory disease row of the table. Fill in the correct answers on Poster 7. Students should fill in the correct answers in their blank Table 3.

Typhoid fever

Typhoid is caused by drinking water or eating food made dirty with human faeces. Patients with typhoid may become very ill after 2 or 3 weeks. Typhoid may damage the bowel and cause peritonitis.

Diagnosis: Typhoid causes a fever which comes and goes. A patient with typhoid usually has a headache, feels tired and is often constipated. He may have a cough.

Treatment: Cross out the box below that does not apply in your country.

In malaria areas

Treat for malaria. If the fever is no better after 5 days, and a blood test shows that the patient does not have malaria, send him to hospital. Typhoid is one cause of a fever which continues for more than a week.

In areas where there is no malaria

Tell the patient to go to hospital if the fever is no better after 5 days.

Ask the students what to write in each space of the typhoid row of the table. Fill in the correct answers on Poster 7. Students should fill in the correct answers in their blank Table 3.

Volvulus

Show the students what happens to the bowel if the patient has volvulus. Use the sock that you have prepared. Hold the two ends of the sock with one hand. Turn the loop of the sock around.

Volvulus is caused when part of the bowel turns around inside the abdomen. This stops faeces and air moving inside the bowel. Volvulus may also stop blood from reaching part of the bowel and cause peritonitis.

Diagnosis: Volvulus causes intermittent abdominal pain, usually in the centre of the abdomen or in area 6, vomiting and a swollen abdomen. A patient with a volvulus does not pass faeces or air.

Treatment: Send a patient who has a painful swollen abdomen immediately to a hospital that does operations.

Ask the students what to write in each space of the volvulus row of the table. Fill in the correct answers on Poster 7. Students should fill in the correct answers in their blank Table 3.

Refreshment break

Gastroenteritis and food poisoning

Gastroenteritis and food poisoning cause irritation inside the bowel. Gastroenteritis and food poisoning cause intermittent pain in the centre of the abdomen and in areas 12 and 6. Patients usually have diarrhoea and may vomit. Other people in the patient's home may have similar symptoms.

Ask the students what to write in each space of the gastroenteritis and food poisoning row of the table. Fill in the correct answers on Poster 7. Students should fill in the correct answers in their blank Table 3.

Constipation

Constipation means that the patient has pain or difficulty in passing faeces. A patient may get constipation if she does not eat enough fruit and vegetables or drink enough fluids.

Diagnosis: Constipation may cause intermittent pain in areas 4, 5 or 6. It can result in tearing of the anus. If a patient has a tear in the anus, there will be a sharp pain every time the patient passes faeces. There may also be blood on the outside of the faeces.

Treatment: Advise a patient with constipation to eat plenty of fruit and vegetables and to drink plenty of fluids. If the patient has pain in the anus, tell her to put vegetable oil in and on the anus every time she passes faeces until the pain has gone. Remind the patient to wash her hands with soap (or ash) and water after she does this.

Ask the students what to write in each space of the constipation row of the table. Fill in the correct answers on Poster 7. Students should fill in the correct answers in their blank Table 3.

Urinary tract infection

Urinary tract infections are caused by bacteria. It is easier for bacteria to get into a woman's bladder than a man's bladder. Bacteria may travel into a woman's bladder after sexual intercourse or during pregnancy.

Ask your students to call out the symptoms of a urinary tract infection. Look for the following answers:

Answer Pain on passing urine

Answer Passing urine more often than usual

Answer Pain in the lower abdomen

The patient may have another illness if she passes urine more often than usual or has blood in her urine:
- If a patient passes urine more often than usual, she may have diabetes

- If a patient passes blood in her urine, she may have schistosomiasis.

Teach the students about diabetes mellitus, using Appendix 16, if diabetes is a problem in your area. Teach students how to interpret urine results if they can do urine microscopy in their health centres. Use Appendix 17.

If the patient is pregnant and you think she has a urinary tract infection, treat with amoxicillin. Give 250 mg three times a day for 5 days. Send patients with a urinary tract infection, schistosomiasis or possible diabetes to hospital.

Ask the students what to write in each space of the urinary tract infection row of the table. Fill in the correct answers on Poster 7. Students should fill in the correct answers in their blank Table 3.

Kidney infection (pyelonephritis)

Sometimes the bacteria that cause a urinary tract infection can infect the kidneys. A patient with a kidney infection has fever and pain in area 3 or 9. He will also have symptoms of a urinary tract infection. Send the patient to hospital.

Ask the students what to write in each space of the kidney infection row of the table. Fill in the correct answers on Poster 7. Students should fill in the correct answers in their blank Table 3.

Kidney stones (stones in a ureter)

Kidney stones are very painful. This problem causes intermittent pain in areas 3 or 9. Give the patient ibuprofen 600 mg three times a day until the pain has gone.
- If the patient is vomiting, put the ibuprofen into her rectum. Tell the patient to drink plenty of fluids. Give the patient 5 ml of fluid every minute if she is vomiting.
- If the patient has vomited four times or more this morning, send her to hospital. This is a general danger sign.
- If the patient also has a fever, treat her for a urinary tract infection.

Ask the students what to write in each space of the kidney stones row of the table. Fill in the correct answers on Poster 7. Students should fill in the correct answers in their blank Table 3.

Hepatitis

Viral hepatitis is the most common cause of jaundice. Viral hepatitis is caused by drinking water or eating food made dirty with human faeces. Jaundice is also caused by severe malaria and by infection with other parasites. Some medicines can cause jaundice. These include medicines for tuberculosis, for psychiatric problems, and paracetamol.

To diagnose jaundice, ask the patient to look upwards. If the white part of his eye is yellow, the patient has jaundice. Only look for jaundice in sunlight. Send all patients with jaundice to hospital immediately.

- If the cause of the jaundice is viral hepatitis, the patient needs no treatment and the jaundice usually improves in 2 weeks. Advise patients with hepatitis to rest, to eat a mixed diet and not to drink alcohol for 3 months.
- If medicines could be the cause of the jaundice, tell the patient to stop taking the medicines.

Ask the students what to write in each space of the hepatitis row of the table. Fill in the correct answers on Poster 7. Students should fill in the correct answers in their blank Table 3.

Rectal prolapse

Rectal prolapse is where the lowest part of the bowel comes out of the anus. Children with malnutrition sometimes develop rectal prolapse if they have diarrhoea or a lot of whipworm.

The first thing to do is to push the rectum back into the anus. Use some vegetable oil to help the rectum slide back in. Next, send the patient to hospital. Tell someone to hold the patient's buttocks together on the way to the hospital to stop the rectal prolapse coming out again.

Ask the students what to write in each space of the rectal prolapse row of the table. Fill in the correct answers on Poster 7. Students should fill in the correct answers in their blank Table 3.

The students can put their completed Table 3 on the wall at their health centre.

SECTION 3: When to refer patients to hospital

Make sure each student has a copy of Appendix 18: 'How to treat a patient with abdominal pain or with blood in the faeces'. Give the students two examples of abdominal problems and show them how to use Appendix 18.

SECTION 4: Practical

Activity

Tell the students that this activity is about how to treat three patients who have abdominal problems. Divide the students into groups of five or six. Give them the following three examples. Tell them to use Table 3 and Appendix 18 to answer the questions about each patient. Give the students 30 minutes. Then ask each group what they think the answers are.

Patient 1

Siti is a 24-year-old woman. She has had constant pain in area 6 for 3 days. Siti has had a fever. She has vomited one time today.

She has pain when she passes urine. The pain is not made worse when she has sexual intercourse. Her last normal period was 2 weeks ago. Siti is able to walk easily. She is not anaemic. Area 6 is tender. There is no guarding and no rebound tenderness.

- What questions are important to ask because she is a woman?
- What illness do you think Siti has?
- How will you treat her?

Patient 2

Peter is 17 years old. He has had pain in his abdomen for 2 days. At first the pain was intermittent in the centre of his abdomen. Now it is constant in areas 7 and 8. He has vomited three times today. He has a fever and is sweaty. Peter walks slowly and bends forward. Peter's abdomen is tender. When you press in areas 7 and 8 you find that he has guarding and rebound tenderness.

- What illness does Peter have?
- How will you treat him?

Patient 3

Mario is 54 years old. He has had constant pain in area 12 of his abdomen for 2 months. The pain gets better when Mario eats. Sometimes he vomits. Mario tells you that he was given aspirin one month ago. His pain gets worse when you press area 12. He does not have guarding or rebound tenderness.

- What was wrong with the treatment that Mario was given one month ago?
- What illness does Mario have?
- How will you treat Mario?

Answers

Ask the students to give their answers. Give them the correct answers:

Patient 1

- When was your last normal period? Does your pain come at the same time as your period? Do you feel pain when you have sexual intercourse?
- A urinary tract infection. She may have malaria.
- Send her to hospital.

Patient 2

- Appendicitis.
- Send him immediately to a hospital where operations are done.

Patient 3

- Do not give aspirin to patients who have abdominal pain. Aspirin can cause peptic ulcers.
- Mario may have a peptic ulcer.
- Send Mario to hospital. Tell him not to take aspirin or ibuprofen, and advise him not to smoke.

SECTION 5: Answers to the quiz

Ask the students to call out the answers to each question in the quiz.

1. Name eight causes of peritonitis.
   Appendicitis
   Perforated peptic ulcer
   Intussusception
   Incarcerated hernia
   Ectopic pregnancy
   Pelvic inflammatory disease
   Typhoid
   Volvulus

2. A patient has abdominal pain. What questions should you ask her?
   - Do you have any **problems when** you **pass urine?**
   - Are your **bowels all right?**
   - **When was** your **last normal** menstrual **period?** Does your **pain** come **at the same time** as your period? Do you feel **pain when** you **have sexual intercourse?**
   - Show me **where** you feel the pain.
   - What type of pain do you feel? Is the pain **constant or intermittent?**
   - Is there **anyone else** at home who has the same symptoms as you?

Lesson 9   Heart problems

BEFORE THE LESSON

- There are five posters in this lesson. (See p. 4 for information on how to use the posters.)
  Prepared poster: 1
  Student answer posters: 2, 5
  Summary posters: 3, 4

- Prepare some example blood pressure measurements so students can practise how to calculate the average blood pressure.

- You need a male student to volunteer to allow you to draw two crosses on his back.

- Give each student a copy of Table 1 'When to refer patients to hospital'.

- For section 4, you need two patients who have heart failure with crackles in both lungs or fluid under the skin in the legs. Ask the patients to meet you in the classroom after the refreshment break. Tell them that you will give them a small payment for coming. Do not forget to bring some money with you to the lesson.

- Show four students how to measure blood pressure. Teach them how to teach this to other students.

- Show four students how to listen to the lower part of both lungs. You will need stethoscopes and equipment for measuring blood pressure.

SECTION 1:   Quiz

POSTER 1:
(Prepared poster)

Quiz
Ask the students to answer the questions on their own. Do not give the answers until the end of the lesson.

> 1. What would you find when you take a history and examine a patient who has heart failure?
> 2. What treatment may save the life of a patient who has had a myocardial infarction?
> 3. What medicine should you give to patients with angina or a cerebrovascular incident?
> 4. Which patients should have their blood pressure measured?
> 5. What advice should you give to people who have high blood pressure?

SECTION 2: Diagnosis and management of heart problems

Heart problems are an important cause of illness and death in all parts of the world. Heart problems are more common in people who smoke.

Today you will learn about three groups of heart problems:
- heart failure
- angina and myocardial infarction
- high blood pressure and the problems caused by high blood pressure.

Heart failure

The heart is a bag of muscle that pushes blood to all parts of the body. Heart failure causes fluid to collect in parts of the body, often in the lungs or lower legs. If you find fluid under the skin in the lower legs, send the patient to hospital immediately.

Fluid in the lungs may cause fast breathing. Remember that patients with pneumonia also have fast breathing.
- If a patient has fast breathing and a fever, treat him for pneumonia. If he is no better after treatment, send him to hospital immediately. He may have heart failure.
- If a patient with fast breathing does not have a fever, listen to his chest. Listen to the lower part of both lungs. If you hear crackles in both lungs, send the patient to hospital immediately. He may have heart failure.

Ask a male student to take off his shirt. Draw two crosses on the student's back 5 cm below the scapulae. Show them how to listen to the chest (Picture 23).

Put the stethoscope in your ears and put the other end on one of the crosses. Ask the patient to breathe in and out deeply. Listen carefully. Listen for a crackling noise. Listen to both sides of the chest. If you can hear a crackling noise on both sides of the chest, the patient has heart failure.

Heart failure can be caused by:
- severe anaemia
- high blood pressure
- myocardial infarction
- tuberculous pericarditis (tuberculosis of the bag around the heart)
- rheumatic heart disease
- congenital heart disease.

Patients with congenital heart disease or rheumatic heart disease are treated with intramuscular benzathine penicillin every 3 weeks for the rest of their life. Give patients who weigh 30 kg or less 0.6 million IU. Give all other patients 1.2 million IU.

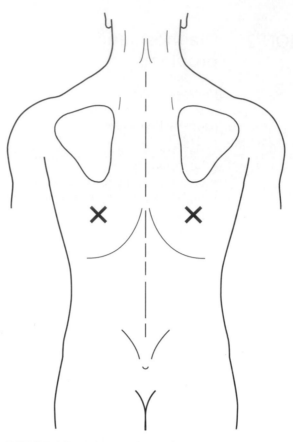

PICTURE 23 *Where to listen for heart failure*

Angina and myocardial infarction

The coronary arteries are tubes that take blood into the heart muscle.

- If the coronary arteries are very narrow, the heart muscle is painful when the patient is moving. This is called angina. Angina pain normally feels like the inside of the chest is being squeezed, crushed or grabbed. The pain of angina is sometimes in the neck or left upper arm. The pain of angina stops when the patient rests. The pain does not last for longer than 20 minutes.

- If the coronary arteries become blocked some of the heart muscle will die. This is called a myocardial infarction, heart attack or MI. The pain of a myocardial infarction is the same as angina pain. The pain of a myocardial infarction normally lasts for more than 20 minutes. Patients who are having a myocardial infarction are often cold, sweaty and anxious. Patients often feel nauseated. They may vomit. Many patients die soon after a myocardial infarction.

Smoking can make the coronary arteries narrow. Usually only people who are more than 40 years old have angina or myocardial infarctions. If you think a patient has had a myocardial infarction give him an aspirin tablet (300 mg) immediately. This will stop some patients from dying.

Send patients who have angina or have had a myocardial infarction to hospital. At hospital the patient may be given other medicines. Give all patients who have angina or have had a myocardial infarction a quarter of a tablet of aspirin (75 mg) every day, for the rest of their lives. Aspirin makes myocardial infarction less likely. Advise these patients to stop smoking. Advise them that regular physical activity (work or exercise) is good, but that they should avoid strenuous exercise if it causes chest pain.

High blood pressure

Blood goes around the body inside tubes called arteries. If these arteries become narrow, the heart has to work harder to push the blood round. You can tell how hard the heart is working by measuring the blood pressure. If the blood pressure is high, the heart is working harder than usual. Another name for high blood pressure is hypertension.

POSTER 2:
(Student answer poster)

Illnesses caused by high blood pressure
Ask the students what illnesses can be caused by high blood pressure.

Answer **Heart failure**

Answer **Myocardial infarction**

Answer **Cerebrovascular incident**. A cerebrovascular incident is also called a stroke or a CVI. A stroke is usually caused when an artery leading to the brain is blocked. If this happens, part of the brain dies. A stroke can cause weakness on one side of the patient's body. It can also cause death. If a patient has had a stroke, giving the patient aspirin can help to stop her having another stroke. Give a quarter of a tablet of aspirin (75 mg) every day for the rest of the patient's life.

Answer **Blindness** or **kidney failure**

Heart failure, myocardial infarction, stroke and kidney failure can kill people. High blood pressure is dangerous. A patient with high blood pressure is two times as likely to die in the next year as a patient with normal blood pressure.

There are two types of blood pressure:
1. the diastolic blood pressure, which is the lower blood pressure
2. the systolic blood pressure, which is the upper blood pressure.

The diastolic blood pressure is more important than the systolic blood pressure. In this manual 'blood pressure' means diastolic blood pressure. If a patient has a diastolic blood pressure of 130 mmHg or more and takes no blood pressure medicine, he will probably die in less than a year.

POSTER 3:	**Four things to prevent illness and death from high blood pressure**
(Summary poster)	

We can do four things to prevent illness and death from high blood pressure:

1. **Check** for high **blood pressure every 5 years** in **all patients aged** more than **45 years**. It is important to measure the blood pressure because patients with high blood pressure usually have no symptoms. Measure the blood pressure if a patient has a severe headache, is aware of his heart beating or if he has poor eyesight.
2. **Give healthy heart advice** to people who have high blood pressure.
3. **Send** a patient who has a diastolic **blood pressure** which is *on average* **105 mmHg or higher, to hospital**.
4. **Make sure** that **patients** who are given medicine for high blood pressure **take** the **medicine** every day.

POSTER 4:	**When to measure blood pressure**
(Summary poster)	

- If the patient has a blood pressure of **120 mmHg or higher, send him to hospital immediately**.
- If a patient has a blood pressure of **95 mmHg or less, measure** the blood pressure **again after 5 years**.
- If the patient has a blood pressure of **less than 120 mmHg but more than 95 mmHg, measure** the blood pressure **again on 3 different days**.
- If the patient is pregnant, measure the blood pressure every **2 weeks in the last 3 months** of the pregnancy.

How to calculate the average blood pressure

Measure a patient's blood pressure on three different days. To calculate the average blood pressure, add up the three blood pressure measurements and divide this number by three. The answer will be the average blood pressure.

Give your students examples of different blood pressure measurements for patients. Ask the students to calculate the average blood pressure for each patient.

Healthy heart advice

Give healthy heart advice to all patients who have a blood pressure of more than 90 mmHg.

POSTER 5:	**Healthy heart advice**
(Student answer poster)	Ask your students what advice they can give to help patients to reduce their blood pressure or to prevent heart problems.

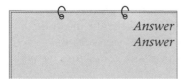

Answer
Answer

Do not smoke.
Do physical work or exercise three times or more **every week** for 20 minutes. This exercise should make the patient sweat but should not cause pain in the chest.

Answer
Answer

Do not add salt to food during cooking or eating.
Eat one banana, or more, **every day** if possible.

Treatment

- If a patient has an average blood pressure of 105 mmHg or more, send him to a high blood pressure clinic. He will take medicine every day for the rest of his life. Hydrochlorothiazide 25 mg once a day, bendroflumethiazide (bendrofluazide) 2.5 mg once a day or atenolol 50 mg once a day are examples. The treatment should reduce the blood pressure to less than 90 mmHg.
- If a patient has an average blood pressure between 95 mmHg and 105 mmHg, do not give medicine to reduce the blood pressure because this will not help the patient.
- If the patient is a pregnant woman, different treatment is needed. See eclampsia and pre-eclampsia in Lesson 7.

SECTION 3: When to refer patients to hospital

Give each student a copy of Table 1.

TABLE 1 When to refer patients to hospital

Heart problem	Symptoms or signs	Treatment
Heart failure	Fast breathing but no fever and has crackles in both lungs. *Or* swelling of ankles, liver, neck or face	Send to hospital immediately
Angina or myocardial infarction	Squeezing pain, crushing pain or grabbing pain in middle of chest. Sometimes in the neck or left upper arm	Give aspirin 300 mg. Send to hospital immediately
High blood pressure All patients	Blood pressure 120 mmHg and above	Send to hospital immediately
	Average blood pressure 105 mmHg and above	Send to clinic for treatment for high blood pressure
Pregnant women	Blood pressure 95–99 mmHg	Send to hospital this week
	Blood pressure 100 mmHg and above	Send to hospital immediately

Refreshment break

SECTION 4: Practical

How to measure blood pressure

Divide the students into four groups. Ask your four student helpers to teach each group how to measure the blood pressure (Picture 24). Each student will practise measuring the blood pressure of another student, who will play the patient.

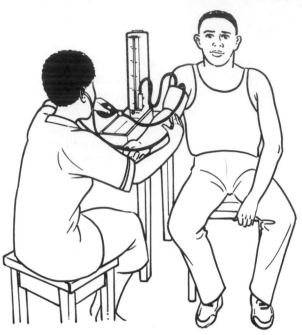

PICTURE 24   *Measuring blood pressure*

1. Ask the patient to sit down. Sometimes the patient can only lie down.
2. Remove all the clothing from the patient's right arm.
3. Put the blood pressure cuff tightly around the upper part of the right arm. Put the cuff at least 2 cm above the bend in the arm. The bladder (inflatable part) of the cuff should cover at least the front part of the arm.
4. The patient's palm should face upwards. Ask him to rest his hand on the table next to him. Put the blood pressure measurement scale on the same table.
5. Put the stethoscope in your ears. Put the other end of the stethoscope on the front of the bend in the arm, on the part that is closest to the patient's body.
6. Turn the valve so that, when you press the rubber bulb, air stays in the cuff. Press the rubber bulb several times until the measurement scale is *above 200 mmHg.*
7. Open the valve slowly, a small amount at a time, until air escapes slowly from the cuff. Listen for a noise each time the heart beats. You will only hear this noise between the top blood pressure (systolic blood pressure) and the bottom blood pressure (diastolic blood pressure).
   - If you do this too quickly you will get the blood pressure wrong.
   - If you do this too slowly you will hurt the patient.
   - If you do this at the correct speed you will hear a noise as the heart beats each time the mercury comes down 4 mmHg.

8. When you hear the first noise look at the top of the mercury or at the needle. Read the number. This is the top blood pressure. When the noise first becomes very quiet or stops, read the number. This is the bottom blood pressure. Write down the two blood pressures: for example, BP 140/90.

   - If the patient is a pregnant women or has a fever or anaemia, the noise becomes *quiet* after you reach the bottom blood pressure.
   - If the patient has high blood pressure, the noise may disappear between 180 mmHg and 160 mmHg. This is *not* the bottom blood pressure. The noise comes back again as the mercury or needle comes down further.

How to look for heart failure

Activity

Now tell the students to divide into two groups and ask the two patients with heart failure to come into the class.
Ask one group to listen for crackles in the lungs and look at the legs of the two patients. Ask the other group to listen for crackles in the lungs and look at the legs of two students. After 10 minutes, change groups. Ask the student helpers to help the groups to listen for the crackles and look for fluid under the skin of the legs of the two patients with heart failure.

SECTION 5:   Answers to the quiz

Ask the students to call out the answers to each question.

1. What would you find when you take a history and examine a patient who has heart failure?
   Fast breathing or fluid under the skin in the legs. You may hear crackles in both lungs.

2. What treatment may save the life of a patient who has had a myocardial infarction?
   Give the patient aspirin 300 mg immediately and 75 mg every day for the rest of his life. Send the patient to hospital.

3. What medicine should you give to patients with angina or a cerebrovascular incident?
   Give aspirin 75 mg every day for the rest of their lives.

4. Which patients should have their blood pressure measured?
   Patients over 45 years: every 5 years
   Patients with a severe headache or who are aware of their heart beating or who have poor eyesight. Pregnant women in the last 3 months of pregnancy.

5. What advice should you give a patient who has high blood pressure?
   - **Do not smoke.**
   - **Exercise three times or more every week for 20 minutes or more.**
   - **Do not add salt to your food when cooking or eating.**
   - **Eat one banana, or more, every day if possible.**

Lesson 10 Accidents, emergencies, joints and the back

BEFORE THE LESSON

- There are 16 posters in this lesson. (See p. 4 for information on how to use the posters.)
  Prepared posters: 1, 8, 11, 12
  Student answer posters: 2, 3, 4, 5, 6, 7, 9, 10, 13, 14, 15, 16. Only write the title on Poster 15 – the students will complete Poster 15 during the lesson. (There are no summary words.)

- Give each student a copy of Appendix 19.

- You need a bed or a table at the front of the class for the role play in section 2. Practise before the lesson.

- Ask one student to help you with the demonstration in section 4. Give the student a copy of the demonstration and practise with her before the lesson.

- For the role play you need clothes, a piece of rope, some leaves, a cup of water, a short stick and piece of cloth.

SECTION 1:   Quiz

POSTER 1:
(Prepared poster)

Quiz
Ask the students to answer the questions on their own. Do not give the answers until the end of the lesson.

> 1. If a patient has been hit on the head, what questions should you ask him?
> 2. What are the main causes of anaphylaxis:
>   - in health centres?
>   - at home?
> 3. What can you do to help a patient who has shock after an accident?
> 4. How will you examine a patient who has a painful knee?

SECTION 2:   Diagnosis and management

Most of today's lesson will be told as a story about *you*. You have finished your training as a primary health care worker. You are working in a health centre. On the first day, you will see many problems which are accidents and emergencies. On the second day, you will see patients who have back or joint problems. On the third day, you will see five patients with back pain.

Accidents and emergencies

Head injuries

On the first day you are cycling to work. You find a man who has driven his car into a mango tree. The man has blood on his head. The man is breathing but he does not answer or move when you shout in his ear.

POSTER 2:
(Student answer poster)

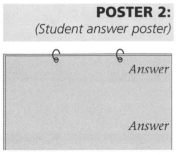

Answer

Answer

How to treat a patient with a head injury
Ask the students what four things they should do for a patient with a head injury.

Do not move the head until you **get help** from two or more people. **Put** the **head in line with** the **body**. Make sure the head cannot move. **Move** the patient **to a safe place**.

As soon as possible, **lay** the patient **on** his **side** in the coma position. This will help him to breathe.

Put a student volunteer into the coma position (Picture 25) in front of the other students.

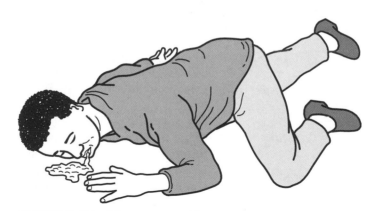

PICTURE 25 *The coma position*

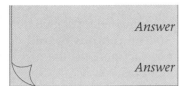

Answer

Answer

Use two fingers to **remove** any **vomit from** his **mouth**. Make sure that his **tongue** is **not at the back of** his **mouth**.

Send the patient to **hospital** with a record card. On the record card write the time of the accident or the time when you found him.

Ask four students to show the class how to treat a patient with a head injury. Tell them what they do correctly and what they could do better.

You continue to cycle to work. You are stopped by Maryam who is worried about her son Tobias. Tobias was hit on his head by a coconut this morning. You need to ask Maryam five questions. If Maryam says 'yes' to any of these questions you must send Tobias to hospital immediately. Tell Maryam to take Tobias to hospital immediately if she can say 'yes' to these questions later in the day or tomorrow.

POSTER 3:
(Student answer poster)

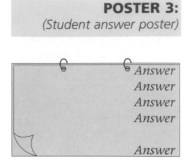

| Answer |
| Answer |
| Answer |
| Answer |
| Answer |

Five questions to ask patients with a head injury
Ask the students which questions to ask patients with a head injury.

1. Did he **lose consciousness** for more than 1 minute?
2. Is it **impossible to wake** him completely?
3. Has he **vomited three times or more**?
4. Has he got a **very painful headache or** a **large wound** on his head?
5. Does he have any **unusual feeling** in his arms or legs?

Cuts

Your first patient at the health centre, Sita, has a large cut on her arm. First, treat the wound. This is similar to treatment for skin ulcers (see Lesson 5). Next, send Sita to hospital to have the wound sewn together. This wound can be sewn together because Sita was injured today and the wound is bigger than 1 cm in size.

POSTER 4:
(Student answer poster)

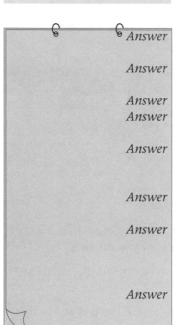

| Answer |
| Answer |
| Answer |
| Answer |
| Answer |
| Answer |
| Answer |
| Answer |

How to treat a wound
Ask the students to tell you how to treat a wound.

1. **Clean the wound**. Use a syringe to squirt normal saline or clean water at the wound.
2. **Cut away** any **black matter**, but do not remove black clotted blood.
3. Put **polyvidone iodine** 10% on the wound.
4. Cover the wound with a **clean dressing**. Put unripe slices of **papaya flesh** underneath the dressing.
5. **Change** the dressing **every 2 days** until the wound is dry. Clean the wound very gently with polyvidone iodine or normal saline.
6. If the wound has been sewn together, **take out** the **stitches after 7 days**.
7. If the patient has not been immunised against tetanus, give her a tetanus vaccination this week. Give 0.5 ml **tetanus toxoid** intramuscularly. Give two more tetanus vaccinations, the first after 1 month and the second after 2 months.
8. Give another tetanus vaccination after 10 years, and another vaccination after another 10 years. A total of five injections will prevent tetanus for life.

Tell your students:

Good wound treatment is very important. Good wound treatment can help to prevent tetanus.

Broken bones

Your next patient, Yusuf, fell out of a tree this morning. He has pain in his right arm and his forearm is bent. You can see that a bone is pressing against the skin. The skin in that place is white.

POSTER 5:
(Student answer poster)

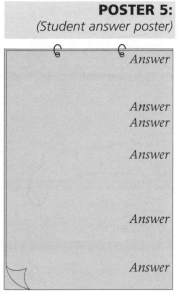

Answer

Answer
Answer

Answer

Answer

Answer

How to treat broken bones
Ask the students: How will you treat Yusuf?

1. If a bone is broken and presses on the skin, **make** the **bone straight** immediately. First, pull both ends of the arm or leg away from the broken bone. Next, make it straight.
2. **If** the **skin** is **broken, cover** the wound **with** a **clean cloth**.
3. **If** the wound is **bleeding heavily**, **press** on the wound **firmly** until the bleeding stops.
4. **If** a **large bone** has been broken, **give** the patient **diazepam** rectally (see Appendix 4). Give the same dose as for treating convulsions. Diazepam reduces anxiety. If available, also give a strong medicine to reduce pain (pethidine for example).
5. **Stop** the arm or leg **from bending** where it is broken. Place a straight stick next to the arm or leg. Tie the arm or leg to the stick with cloth.
6. **Send** a patient who has a **broken large bone to hospital** immediately.

Show the students Picture 26 of how to make a broken bone straight.

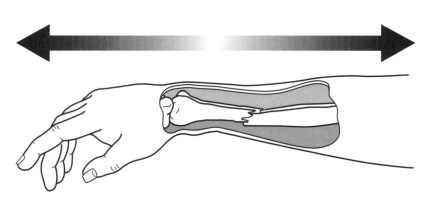

PICTURE 26 *How to make a broken bone straight*

Ask two students to help you. Ask one to play a patient with a broken arm. Ask the other student to pull the arm at the elbow. You will pull at the wrist.

Show the students Picture 27 of how to stop a broken leg from bending.

Ask the students: If a patient has broken a bone but the bone is not bent, how can we tell that it is broken? Look for the following answer:

Answer If a bone is broken it will be painful when you push the ends of that bone together.

135

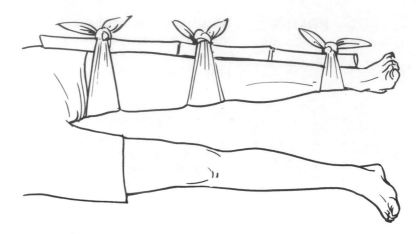

PICTURE 27 *How to stop a broken leg from bending*

Shock

Shock means that not enough blood reaches the brain and other parts of the body. Shock is very dangerous. Patients with shock may become unconscious or die.

Shock may be caused by:
- blood loss and broken bones
- anaphylaxis, which is a severe allergic reaction.

Tell the students that the heart beats fast in shock. Feel one of the arteries in the neck to count how many times the heart beats in 1 minute. Show the students where to feel. The movement of the arteries is called the pulse.

Hamida, your next patient, has broken her leg bone. Hamida feels light-headed. She tells you that she feels as if she might faint. She is sweating and cold. Her pulse is weak and faster than 110 beats in one minute. Hamida has shock caused by blood loss and a broken bone.

POSTER 6:
(Student answer poster)

How to treat shock from blood loss and broken bones
Ask the students: How will you treat Hamida?

How to treat shock from blood loss and broken bones

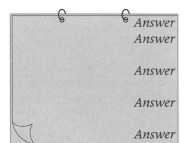

Answer
Answer

Answer

Answer

Answer

- **Treat** the cause of the **shock**. **Stop** the **bleeding** if possible.
- Place a stick next to the broken arm or leg and **tie** the **stick to the arm or leg** with cloth.
- **Give** the patient **rectal diazepam** if she has broken a large bone.
- **Give** the patient **oral rehydration solution**. Give her 5 ml (1 teaspoon) every minute.
- **Send** the patient **to hospital** immediately.

Anaphylaxis

Next, the orderly calls for your help. He has just given a 24-year-old man an injection of procaine penicillin fortified. The patient has lost consciousness and is cold and sweaty. His pulse is weak and faster than 110 beats in 1 minute. The patient has shock caused by anaphylaxis.

There are three common causes of anaphylaxis:
- medicines – antibiotic injections, antibiotic tablets or vaccinations may cause anaphylaxis
- food – some people are allergic to some foods, for example nuts, prawns or squid
- insect bites and stings – usually from bees and spiders.

POSTER 7:
(Student answer poster)

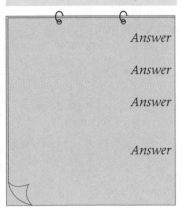

Answer

Answer

Answer

Answer

How to treat anaphylaxis
Ask the students: How will you treat this patient?

To treat a patient with anaphylaxis:
1. Give him an injection of **epinephrine** (also called adrenaline), 1 in 1000, **intramuscularly**.
2. Give a **second** injection of epinephrine **after 10 minutes** if the patient is still unconscious or has a fast pulse.
3. **If** the patient is **still** unconscious or **unwell** 10 minutes after the second injection of epinephrine, **give** him a **third injection** of epinephrine. **Send** him **to hospital** immediately.
4. When the patient is well, **tell him** that **he has an allergy**. Tell the patient what he is allergic to, if you know. Teach the patient and the patient's family that in future he must avoid the thing he is allergic to.

Tell your students: The dose of epinephrine is different for patients of different ages.

POSTER 8:
(Prepared poster)

Doses of epinephrine
Copy Table 1 onto Poster 8.

TABLE 1   Doses of epinephrine

Age of patient	Dose of epinephrine	
Up to 12 months	0.1 ml	–
1 year up to 5 years	0.25 ml	$\frac{1}{4}$ vial
5 years old or more	0.5 ml	$\frac{1}{2}$ vial

Kerosene poisoning

Gabriel, your last patient of the day, is a 3-year-old boy. Gabriel has drunk some kerosene. To treat a patient who has drunk kerosene:
1. Send the patient to hospital.
2. Tell the patient to drink lots of young coconut juice or water on the way to hospital.
3. *Do not* make the patient vomit.

Rabies

On your way home you pass through Kijini village. Earlier today the villagers killed a dog which had bitten two people. The villagers thought the dog had rabies.

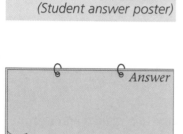

POSTER 9:
(Student answer poster)

How to treat patients with bites from an animal with rabies

Ask the students what they should do for patients who are bitten by animals that may have rabies

Answer

1. **Wash wounds immediately**. The best cleaning fluids are iodine or alcohol. Iodine and alcohol kill viruses. However, water, with or without soap, will help. Even urine is better than nothing. Use a brush to clean the wound if possible.

Answer

2. **Send** the two patients **to hospital** immediately.

Burns

At home, your neighbour brings her 6-year-old son Raju to you. Raju has burnt himself. A large pan of hot water fell on his abdomen and the front of his right leg.

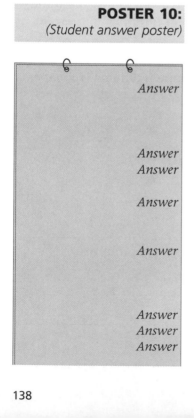

POSTER 10:
(Student answer poster)

Immediate treatment for burns

Ask the students: How will you treat Raju?

Immediate treatment for burns

Answer

1. **Wash** and cool the burn **with cold water**. Hold the part of the body that has been burnt underneath a running tap for about 20 minutes or in a bucket of cold water for the same length of time.

Answer

2. Do **not** break any blisters.

Answer

3. If the burn is dirty, clean it gently with normal saline or polyvidone iodine 10%.

Answer

4. Put **unripe papaya flesh** on the burn. This is a very good antiseptic. It helps the burnt skin to heal and also stops the skin sticking to the cloth.

Answer

5. If you have no papaya, paint the wound with **gentian violet**. Next, put some **vaseline, or vegetable fat which has been boiled and cooled**, on the burn to stop the skin sticking to the cloth.

Answer

6. **Cover** the burn **with** a **clean cloth**.

Answer

7. **Change** the dressings **every 2 days**.

Answer

8. Make sure that the patient has been immunised against tetanus. If not, give him **tetanus toxoid** as soon as possible.

Answer

Answer

Answer

9. **You do not** normally need to **give** an **antibiotic** to a patient who has a burn.
10. **If** the **burn** becomes **covered** with yellow or green **pus, smells bad or** is getting **bigger:**
    - clean the wound again
    - dress the wound with papaya, or gentian violet and vaseline
    - treat the patient with **co-trimoxazole** for 5 days.
11. If the burn has **not started to heal after 1 week** send him to hospital.

Degree of the burn

To decide whether a patient needs to go to hospital you need to know:
- the degree of the burn
- the percentage of the skin area that has been burned.

POSTER 11:
(Prepared poster)

Answer

Answer

Answer

The three degrees of burns

The **degree of** the **burn is** the **depth of** the **burn**. There are three degrees of burn:

1. **First-degree** burns only affect the very **outside layer** of the skin. The skin is **red** and **tender**.
2. **Second-degree** burns affect the **outside and middle layers** of the skin. The skin becomes **blistered** and **tender**.
3. **Third-degree** burns affect the **outside, middle and bottom layers** of skin. There is no blistering of the skin in that area. The skin may be **black or white**. The skin has no feeling and is **not tender**. The skin is not able to grow back in a third-degree burn.

A patient with third-degree burns needs to go to hospital.

Percentage of skin

If a patient burns a large percentage of his skin area, he will lose a large amount of fluid and will get infections. Patients with burns should drink plenty of fluids.

Dehydration and infections may kill the patient.

A patient who has burnt 10% or more of his skin area needs to go to hospital.

A patient who has a burn on his face or private parts also needs to go to hospital.

POSTER 12:
(Prepared poster)

Percentages of skin area of each part of the body of a child and of an adult

Draw Pictures 28 and 29 on Poster 12.

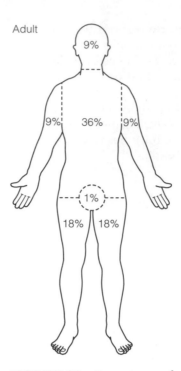

Adult

9%

9% 36% 9%

1%

18% 18%

PICTURE 28 *Percentages of skin area which cover each part of the body of an adult*

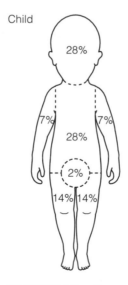

Child

28%

7% 7%

28%

2%

14% 14%

PICTURE 29 *Percentages of skin area which cover each part of the body of a child who is less than 12 years old*

Pictures 28 and 29 show the percentages of the skin area that cover each part of the body of an adult and a child aged 12 years or less.

For example:

- The skin that covers the leg of a child is 14% of the total skin area. If a child burnt only the front of one leg, he would have a 7% burn.
- The skin that covers the whole of the chest together with the abdomen of an adult is 36% of the total skin area. In a child the same area is 28% of the total skin area. If an adult burnt only the front of the abdomen, he would have a 9% burn (a quarter of 36%). If a child burns only the front of the abdomen, he would have a 7% burn (a quarter of 28%).

Give the students three examples of patients who have burnt parts of the body. Ask the students to calculate the area of skin burnt on each patient. Show them how to work this out using Raju as an example:

Raju has burnt all of the front of his abdomen. This is 7% of his total skin area. Raju has also burnt the front of his right leg. This is 7% of his total skin area (half of 14%). In total, Raju has burnt 14% of his skin area. Send Raju to hospital for further treatment.

Refreshment break.

Joints and the back

On your second day at work, you see patients with joint and back problems.

Arthritis

Your first patient today is a 47-year-old man called Max. Max's knee has been painful and swollen for 4 days. You ask Max if the knee was injured. Max cannot remember hurting his knee. You ask Max if he has a fever. Max tells you that he has been hot and sweaty at night for 4 days.

POSTER 13:
(Student answer poster)

Answer

Answer
Answer

Answer

Things to look for in patients with joint pain
Ask the students what four things to look for if a patient has joint pain.

1. Look to see if the joint is more **swollen** than the joint on the other side.
2. Feel to see if the joint is more **hot** than the rest of the body.
3. Press the swelling to find out if it is soft or hard and bony. Ask the patient if the joint is **tender**.
4. Ask the patient to **bend** the joint. Ask him if it is **more painful** when he bends the joint.

A patient with arthritis has pain and swelling of one or many joints. Arthritis causes patients to have permanent and often increasing difficulty in using their joints. Arthritis is divided into two types: septic arthritis and other types of arthritis. The patient may have any of these types of arthritis.

Septic arthritis

Septic arthritis must be treated immediately. If the patient has not been injured and has a soft, hot or tender swelling in one joint, and bending the joint is very painful, the patient has septic arthritis. Max's knee has soft, tender swelling but does not feel hot. It is painful to bend his knees. He may have septic arthritis.

Send patients with septic arthritis to hospital immediately. If it will take longer than 6 hours for the patient to get to the hospital, give co-trimoxazole at twice the normal dose.

Other types of arthritis

Diagnose other types of arthritis if a patient has had pain for more than 6 weeks with hard or soft swelling around one or more joints. The most common other types of arthritis are osteoarthritis and rheumatoid arthritis.

If a patient has rheumatoid arthritis, he has swelling in the joints on **both** sides of the body. Two different joints **and** the joints in the hands will be swollen. The swelling is soft and may be warm and tender. Send patients with possible rheumatoid arthritis to see a joint expert (a rheumatologist) if possible.

- Treat other types of arthritis with paracetamol: two tablets four times a day. Tell the patient not to take more paracetamol than this dose. Higher doses can damage the liver.
- If paracetamol is not helpful, give ibuprofen 600 mg three times a day after food. Tell patients to stop taking ibuprofen if they get pain at the top of the abdomen. Advise the patient to bend and straighten each joint several times every day.

Osteomyelitis

Marcelle, your next patient, has pain in his upper leg, not in his joint. Marcelle has not had an accident. Marcelle cannot walk. The bone is tender. The upper leg is hot. Marcelle has osteomyelitis. Osteomyelitis is an infection of bone. Give Marcelle twice the normal dose of co-trimoxazole and send him immediately to hospital.

Diagnosing and treating patients with back pain

Five patients with common and important types of back pain come to your health centre today. Your job is to decide which type of back problem each patient has.

POSTER 14:
(Student answer poster)

Seven questions for patients with back pain
Ask the students which seven questions we need to ask patients to find out the cause of back pain.

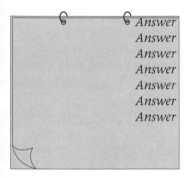

Answer
Answer
Answer
Answer
Answer
Answer
Answer

1. **How long** have you had back pain?
2. Have you had a bad fall or an **accident**?
3. Is the pain **worse after exercise**?
4. Is the pain **constant**?
5. Do you have a **fever**?
6. Is it **painful when** you **press** on a **bone** in the spine?
7. Ask the patient to lie on his back. Lift one leg at the hip but keep the knee straight. Do the same with the other leg. Ask the patient if there is **pain in** the **back and below the knee when** you **lift the leg**.

Give each student a copy of Appendix 19. Explain to the students that Appendix 19 summarises what they need to know to diagnose the cause of back pain.

Role plays

Tell your students that you will now role-play seven patients. Tell the students to ask you each of the seven questions.
- For question 6, ask a student to press on your spine bones.
- For question 7, lie on your back and ask a student to lift each leg as described above.
- When you role-play patient 3, tell the student that you feel pain in the back and below the knee when she lifts your leg.

Next, ask the students to tell you the diagnosis. Tell the students the treatment.

ROLE PLAY 1:

Patient 1 has had back pain for less than 2 weeks. The pain is often worse after exercise. She has a fever.

Diagnosis: The cause of back pain is fever. Fever causes pain in the muscles of the back.

Treatment: Treat the patient for malaria if there is malaria in the area.

ROLE PLAY 2:

Patient 2 has back pain that gets worse after exercise and gets better after rest.

Diagnosis: The cause of back pain is the back muscles working too hard.

Treatment: Show the patient Show to keep her back straight and bend her knees when bending over. Regular stretching exercises each morning and night will help. Paracetamol is also helpful.

ROLE PLAY 3:

Patient 3 has pain in the lower back. The pain goes down one leg below the knee when the hip is bent.
(Tell the student that you feel pain in the back and below the knee when she lifts your leg.)

Diagnosis: The cause of back pain is a disc prolapse. A disc prolapse happens when the gristle (soft part) between the bones in the spine is damaged and pushed out from between the bones of the spine. Sometimes this gristle is pushed against a nerve. This causes the pain of a disc prolapse.

Treatment: Tell the patient not to work for 2 weeks. He should start doing regular stretching exercises as soon as he can. Give him paracetamol. Refer him to the orthopaedic clinic if the pain has not started to reduce after 2 weeks.

ROLE PLAY 4:

Patient 4 has had pain in the back for more than six weeks. The pain is constant. There is also pain when you press one of the bones in the spine. There may be a fever.

Diagnosis: The cause of back pain is tuberculosis of the spine.

Treatment: Send the patient to the tuberculosis clinic.

ROLE PLAY 5:

Patient 5 has had a bad fall or an accident. There is pain when you press one of the bones in the spine.

Diagnosis: The cause of back pain is a broken bone.

Treatment: Tell the patient to rest completely for 6 weeks. Give her paracetamol. If the patient does not rest she may damage the nerve in her spine. If she damages the nerve in her spine, she may never be able to walk again. If the patient has weakness in her legs or cannot feel part of her legs or around her anus, send her to hospital immediately.

SECTION 3: When to refer patients to hospital

POSTER 15:
(Student answer poster)

When to send patients to hospital
Write the title only on Poster 15 before the lesson.

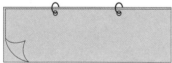

Ask students to write reasons for sending a patient to the hospital on Poster 15. Tell students which of the answers they have written on Poster 15 are correct. Circle the correct answers on Poster 15 so all the students can see them. Look for the following answers:

Answer   • if a patient with a head injury says 'yes' to any of the five questions

Answer   • if a large bone has been broken

Answer   • if a patient has shock caused by blood loss or broken bones

Answer   • if a patient has shock caused by anaphylaxis and is still unconscious or unwell after the second injection of epinephrine

Answer   • if a patient has drunk kerosene

Answer   • if a patient is bitten by an animal that may have rabies

Answer   • if a patient has third-degree burns or burns on more than 10% of the total skin area; if the patient has a burn on the face or private parts or a burn has not started to heal after 1 week

Answer   • if a patient has possible septic arthritis

Answer • if a patient has possible osteomyelitis

Answer • if a patient with a disc prolapse is no better after 2 weeks (send to the orthopaedic clinic)

Answer • if a patient has had constant back pain for 6 weeks or more and part of the spine is tender (send to the TB clinic)

Answer • if the patient has had an accident and has weakness in his legs or cannot feel part of his legs or around his anus

SECTION 4: Practical

Tell the students that this demonstration will show them how to treat snake bites. You need clothes, a piece of rope to represent the snake, some leaves, a cup of water, a short stick and three pieces of cloth. Ask one student to play the woman who is bitten by the snake. You will play the farmer. Practise the demonstration with the student before the lesson.

Demonstration

Woman: Ahhhh ... I've been bitten by a dangerous snake!
Farmer: *Do not worry, snakes are not very good at injecting poison into people. Most snakes do not make dangerous poison.*
Woman: That's nice to know.
Farmer: *Lie down and let me wipe the bite with a piece of cloth.*
Woman: Thank you.
Farmer: *I will wrap a cloth firmly but **not** tightly around the leg. Next, I'm going to stop your leg from moving. I will tie a stick next to the leg.*
Woman: You are very kind.
Farmer: *I will take you to hospital.*
Woman: Thank you sir.

Snake bites usually happen at night, when people walk barefoot and accidentally stand on a snake. Different types of snake cause different types of damage but most snake bites are not dangerous. The damage caused by a snake bite depends on the type of snake and the amount of poison injected. Usually the snake is only able to inject a small amount of poison.

POSTER 16: **How to treat snake bites**
(Student answer poster) Ask the students how to treat snake bites.

Answer 1. **Wipe** the **bite** with a piece of cloth. If the snake spat in the patients' eyes, **wash** the **eyes** thoroughly with water. Even urine will help if there is no water available. Do not cut the bite.

Answer 2. Tell the patient **not to worry**. Snakes are not very good at injecting poison into people. Most snakes do not make dangerous poison.

145

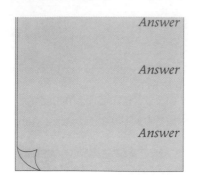

Answer

Answer

Answer

3. Wrap a cloth firmly, but not tightly, around the bitten leg or arm. Stop the bitten leg (or arm) **from moving**. Tie a stick next to the leg.

4. **Send** the patient **to hospital**. If the snake has already been killed, take it to the hospital together with the patient. If the snake is not dead, leave the snake alone. Remember that even a dead snake can still inject poison.

5. **If** the patient **vomits, turn her on her side**. This will prevent the patient from choking on her vomit.

SECTION 5: Answers to the quiz

Ask the students to call out the answers to each question in the quiz.

1. If a patient has been hit on the head, what questions are useful?
   - **Did he lose consciousness for more than 1 minute?**
   - **Is it impossible to wake him completely?**
   - **Has he vomited three times or more?**
   - **Has he got a very painful headache or a large wound to his head?**
   - **Does he have any unusual feeling in his arms or legs?**

2. What are the main causes of anaphylaxis?
   - **Medicines – antibiotic injections, antibiotic tablets and vaccinations**
   - **Foods – some people are allergic to some foods, for example, nuts, prawns or squid**
   - **Insect bites and stings – usually from bees and spiders**

3. What should you do to help a patient who has shock because of an accident?
   - **Treat the cause of the shock. Stop the bleeding if possible.**
   - **Give the patient oral rehydration solution. Give him 1 teaspoon (5 ml) of solution every minute.**
   - **If a large bone has been broken give the patient diazepam rectally. Place a stick next to the arm or leg and tie the stick to the arm or leg with cloth.**
   - **Send the patient to hospital immediately.**

4. If the patient has a painful knee, how will you examine it?
   - **Look to see if the joint is more swollen than the joint on the other side.**
   - **Feel to see if the joint is more hot than the rest of the body.**
   - **Press the swelling to find out if it is soft or hard and bony. Is the joint tender?**
   - **Ask the patient to bend the joint. Is it more painful?**

Lesson 11 | Psychiatric problems

BEFORE THE LESSON

■ There are seven posters in this lesson. (See p. 4 for information on how to use the posters.)
Prepared posters: 1, 3, 5
Student answer posters: 2, 4, 6, 7

■ There are five demonstrations in this lesson. Ask ten students to help you perform the demonstrations. Give each student a copy of the demonstration and ask them to practise the demonstration before the lesson. They may want to dress up for the demonstration.

■ You need a mat or a rug for the first demonstration and some farming tools for the second demonstration.

■ Cross out the box about sleeping sickness if there is no sleeping sickness in your area.

■ For section 4, try to find a traditional healer who is effective at treating anxiety and depression. Ask him if he will teach your students. Tell him that your students may send patients with anxiety and depression to him if they know that he can help them.

SECTION 1: Quiz

POSTER 1: **Quiz**
(Prepared poster) Ask the students to answer the questions on their own. Do not give the answers until the end of the lesson.

> 1. A patient is brought to you because he has been doing strange things for the past 5 days. He does not have a fever.
>   • What questions should you ask to find out if he has severe mental illness?
>   • Where should you send him if you think he has severe mental illness?
> 2. What are the important symptoms of depression?
> 3. What advice should you give to a patient who has epilepsy?

SECTION 2: Diagnosis and management

Tell the students that this lesson will tell them how to help patients with psychiatric problems.

A patient has psychiatric problems when his mind and spirit are ill. There are many causes of psychiatric problems. Health workers need to understand the local culture to be able to help a patient who has an illness of the mind and spirit. Culture means the beliefs and habits that are normal in the patient's community.

Traditional healers often treat patients with psychiatric problems. Traditional healers often know more about patients' culture than health workers. They are often good at treating illnesses like anxiety and depression. Later in the lesson we will hear from a traditional healer about how he treats these illnesses.

We will now talk about several patients with psychiatric problems: severe mental illness, depression and anxiety. You will also learn about epilepsy. Epilepsy is not a psychiatric illness. It is sometimes caused by damage to the brain.

In areas with sleeping sickness: tell your students that they will also learn about sleeping sickness.

Severe mental illness

A patient has severe mental illness if he has one or more of these symptoms:
- hallucinations
- delusions
- thinking in a very unusual or disorganised way.

Patients with severe mental illness can also have symptoms of depression and anxiety. The symptoms of depression and anxiety are discussed later in this section.

POSTER 2:
(Student answer poster)

Answer

Answer

Answer

Questions for all psychiatric patients
Ask your students to tell you what they should do if they think a patient may have a psychiatric illness.

Ask: When you are **on your own**, do you hear peoples' **voices?** Do you often **see things** that are unusual (hallucinations)?

Ask: Do you have any **ideas** that **other people know are not true** that **you know are correct** (delusions)?

Listen: **Listen** to **what** the **patient says**. If what he says **does not make sense** to you, his thoughts may be unusual or disorganised.

Ask: Have you been **sad** for **more than 2 weeks**?

The answers to these questions will tell you whether a patient has a severe mental illness or possible depression.

There are many causes of severe mental illness (sometimes called psychosis). Severe mental illness may be caused by an illness of the body or by a psychiatric illness. Illnesses of the body can sometimes affect the brain and cause mental illness. Illnesses of the body usually last for a short time and can often be cured. Psychiatric illnesses usually last for a long time. Treatment can make psychiatric illnesses better but often the problem will come back again.

POSTER 3:
(Prepared poster)

Common causes of severe mental illness

Illnesses of the body:
- alcohol withdrawal
- cerebral malaria
- meningitis
- head injury
- alcohol intoxication

Psychiatric illnesses:
- schizophrenia
- mania

Demonstrations

Explain to the students that they will now see three demonstrations which will help them remember how to diagnose different causes of severe mental illness. The demonstrations show patients with an illness of the body, with schizophrenia and with mania.

DEMONSTRATION 1:

An illness of the body

Ask one student to play the husband and one to play the wife. You need a mat or rug for this demonstration.

A 20-year-old man is sitting on a mat on the floor. He is restless, shouts and looks anxious. His wife is kneeling next to him and tries to comfort him.

Husband:	*Get those things away from me!*
Wife:	What things?
Husband:	*Those nasty little hairy animals!* (Points to the corner of the room.)
Wife:	I cannot see any animals.

Ask your students to tell you which of the symptoms of severe mental illness this man has. Look for the following answer:

Answer: The man is having hallucinations.

Tell your students:

This man works at the local sugar plantation. He normally spends most of his wages on alcohol. This week the bar has no alcohol so he has had no alcohol to drink. This man is ill with alcohol withdrawal. If someone drinks large amounts of alcohol regularly and then suddenly stops drinking alcohol, he may become ill with alcohol withdrawal. This causes the person to become anxious, shaky and to have convulsions. Give him diazepam 10–20 mg by mouth, or rectally or by intramuscular injection. Give him 50 ml of sugar water or milk. Next, send the patient to hospital.

Alcohol intoxication, alcohol withdrawal, cerebral malaria, meningitis and a head injury are all illnesses of the body that can cause severe mental illness.

Tell the students how to treat a patient with symptoms of severe mental illness:

- If the patient has symptoms of severe mental illness and has been hit on the head, send him to hospital immediately.
- If the patient has symptoms of severe mental illness and has a fever, treat him for very severe febrile disease (see Chapter 2) and send him to hospital immediately.
- If a patient has symptoms of severe mental illness, but does not have fever and has not been hit on the head, send him to see a psychiatric nurse or doctor.

DEMONSTRATION 2: **Schizophrenia**

Ask one student to play the role of the boy and another student to play the role of his mother. You need two farming tools for this demonstration.

A 16-year-old boy and his mother are talking to each other as they farm.

Mother:	*Why don't you talk to other people, Hassan?*
Boy:	The voices tell me not to.
Mother:	*What voices?*
Boy:	The voices that tell me that the people in our village are against me.
Mother:	*But Hassan, the people in the village like you. Where do these voices come from?*
Boy:	I hear the voices in my head when there is nobody there. I know that the people from the village hate me. They want to kill me.
Mother:	*Hassan, the people in the village are very worried about you. You have been behaving very strangely for the last few months. The people in the village do not want to kill you.*
Boy:	I know they do want to kill me. Nothing you can say will stop me knowing that!

Ask your students to tell you which of the symptoms of severe mental illness this boy has. Look for the following answer:

Answer   The boy is having hallucinations, he is hearing voices. The boy has delusions. He thinks the people in his village want to kill him. The people in his village do not want to kill him but the boy knows that he is correct. The boy has thoughts that are unusual.

Ask your students what could cause this boy's severe mental illness. Explain what is wrong with the boy.

This boy does not drink alcohol. He has not been hit on the head. He does not have a fever. The boy is ill with a type of severe mental illness called schizophrenia. A person with schizophrenia cannot tell the difference between things that really do happen and things that do not happen. He may hear voices when there is nobody there. He may feel that he has no control over his thoughts or actions. For example, a patient with schizophrenia may say 'Someone is putting thoughts into my head.' A person can be ill with schizophrenia for many years. The illness sometimes gets better for long periods of time. Other worries can make the schizophrenia worse.

This boy needs to see a psychiatric nurse or doctor. He may need treatment with an antipsychotic medicine. Antipsychotic medicines reduce hallucinations, delusions and abnormal thoughts. Chlorpromazine, haloperidol, thioridazine, trifluoperazine and fluphenazine are examples of antipsychotic medicines. These medicines can cause side effects. One side effect of antipsychotic medicines is acute dystonia.
    The symptoms of acute dystonia are:
- the patient is suddenly unable to turn his neck away from one side
- the patient is unable to look ahead with his eyes
- the patient is unable to open his mouth.

If you think that a patient has acute dystonia, stop the medicine. Next, give trihexyphenidyl (benzhexol) 2 mg three times a day until the symptoms have stopped. Treatment for 3 days is usually enough. Send the patient to see a psychiatric doctor or nurse, who may give the patient a different medicine.

DEMONSTRATION 3:	**Mania**

Ask one student to play the policeman and one to play the woman.

A policeman has been called to the market place. A woman is annoying the sellers at the market. She is talking quickly in a loud voice.

Woman: I tell you all. I am God's messenger. God has brought me back from the dead to set you free from your difficult lives. Come with me now and I will show you all the promised land. I will help you all.

Policeman: *Come with me, madam.*

Woman: Ah officer, I'm glad you came. I've been telling these good people how I can help them. Take me to the radio station so that I can talk to more people. I have a very important job to do. God himself has told me what to do.

Policeman:	*So you are a priest of the church?*
Woman:	Officer, I am the woman who will do God's work on earth. I need no help from the church. I will make the earth a perfect place to live in. All people will soon be as happy as I am.

Ask your students to tell you which of the symptoms of severe mental illness this woman has. Look for the following answer:

Answer:	This woman is having delusions. Her thoughts are unusual.

Ask your students what could be the cause of this woman's illness. Explain what is wrong with her.

This woman does not drink alcohol. She has not been hit on the head and does not have a fever. The woman is ill with a problem called mania.

Tell the students the signs of mania and what to do for a patient with mania.

Patients with mania may:
- be very happy for a long time
- eat a lot and speak quickly
- want to have sex often
- spend all of their money
- think that they are very important
- have hallucinations.

Many patients who have mania some of the time have depression at other times.
Send this woman to see a psychiatric doctor or nurse, who may prescribe an antipsychotic medicine or carbamazepine.

Depression and anxiety

Many things that happen in life can cause anxiety and depression. For example, getting married, taking exams or a serious illness in the family, can make people anxious. People who are anxious for a long time may become ill with depression. Depression can also be caused by a big life event or a problem that continues for a long time. For example, the death of a husband or wife or child can make someone ill with depression.

Ask your students what might cause a patient to be anxious or to become ill with depression.

Demonstrations

Tell the students that they will see two demonstrations about patients with symptoms of depression and anxiety.

DEMONSTRATION 4:

Depression

Ask one student to play the role of a 35-year-old woman, and one to play the role of a traditional healer.

A 35-year-old woman is talking to the traditional healer. Her husband and her son have died in the last 2 months.

Traditional healer:	Tell me how I can help you.
Woman:	*I feel very sad. I cannot sleep and I cry all the time.*
Traditional healer:	I heard about the deaths of your husband and son. I am sorry. Are you able to eat?
Woman:	*No.*
Traditional healer:	What time do you wake up in the morning?
Woman:	*Four o'clock, long before the sun comes up.*
Traditional healer:	Are you able to do your work? Do you do the things that you normally enjoy?
Woman:	*No, I have no interest in anything.*
Traditional healer:	Have you thought about harming yourself?
Woman:	*Yes, but I could not do it. I still have four children to look after.*
Traditional healer:	I can help you get better. You must come to talk to me about how you are feeling every week.

It is normal for people to feel sad some of the time and happy at other times. Talking to a friend or relative about their problems can help most people who are sad. If a person is very sad for longer than 2 weeks and also has three other symptoms, she has depression.

Tell the students again that *all* patients who have depression are very sad for 2 weeks or more.

POSTER 4:
(Student answer poster)

Extra symptoms of depression
Ask your students what the additional symptoms of depression are.

Answer
Answer
Answer
Answer
Answer
Answer
Answer

The patient:

is **not interested in eating**

wakes very early, well before sunrise

is **more sad in the morning** than in the evening

has **no interest** in sexual intercourse or other things that she normally enjoys

is **unable to** do her **work**

thinks that **she is no good** or feels bad for doing something wrong, although she has not done anything wrong

hopes to die or **plans to kill herself.**

Send a patient to see a psychiatric doctor or nurse if she is very sad and also has three or more of these extra symptoms or is planning to kill herself. The psychiatric doctor or nurse may treat depression with counselling or with antidepressant tablets.

Anxiety

Anxiety can cause different symptoms. The symptoms of anxiety include:
- being aware of your heartbeat
- headache
- sweats
- fast breathing
- tingling in the lips and fingers.

But other illnesses can also cause these symptoms. You should look first for fever or anaemia and for symptoms of severe mental illness or depression. If the patient has none of these problems, he probably has anxiety.

If you think a patient has anxiety, ask him what his problems are. Help him to think about his problems and how to solve them himself. Tell the patient that his symptoms are caused by anxiety. Help *the patient* to decide what *he* can do to reduce his problems. This is called counselling. Suggest that the patient talks about his problem with his family or friends to reduce anxiety.

Diazepam should not normally be used to treat anxiety. Diazepam can make the anxiety worse.

DEMONSTRATION 5:

Ask one student to play the role of a 17-year-old woman and one to play the role of a doctor.

The woman is talking to the doctor. She is sitting on the edge of her chair. She is looking down and playing with her fingers.

Doctor: Good morning.

Woman: *Good morning.*

Doctor: How can I help you?

Woman: *I have a headache and I can feel my heart beat.*

Doctor: Anything else?

Woman: *I feel like I'm going to vomit.*

Doctor: Do you have a fever?

Woman: *No.*

Doctor: Do you have a cough?

Woman: *No.*

Doctor: Have you vomited or do you have diarrhoea?

Woman: *No.*

Doctor: What medicine have you used?

Woman: *Just paracetamol.*

Tell your students: The doctor examines the patient. He finds that she is not anaemic and that she does not have a fever. The woman's blood pressure is 110/65.

Doctor:	Headaches, feeling your heart beat and feeling as if you are going to vomit are often caused by worry. Is there anything that is worrying you?
Woman:	… (slowly) … *Well … yes, there is. I was married last month. I did not want to get married.*
Doctor:	I'm sorry. Are you unhappy all the time?
Woman:	*No, I still enjoy meeting my friends.*
Doctor:	Are you sleeping well?
Woman:	*Not bad. It takes a long time to get off to sleep. I do not wake up until sunrise.*
Doctor:	Are you able to eat?
Woman:	*Yes.*
Doctor:	From talking to you and examining you, I can tell you that you do not have any bad illness. Worry or anxiety causes your symptoms. Can you talk to someone else about your worries? It may help to talk to a friend who was also married but did not want to marry. If you are not feeling better in 4 weeks, come to see me again.

How to identify psychiatric problems

Explain to the students that the next story will help them to remember to look for symptoms of severe mental illness in patients who have symptoms of depression or anxiety. It will also help them to remember to look for symptoms of depression in patients who have symptoms of anxiety.

POSTER 5:
(Prepared poster)

Treat the most important psychiatric problem first
Draw Picture 30 (see p. 156) on Poster 5.
Tell the students about the picture:

A fisherman catches three fish to sell at the market in a town 10 km away. The fisherman can only carry one fish on his bicycle. He must choose which fish to take to town. He will be paid the best price for the biggest fish, so he takes the biggest fish with him to sell at the market. He leaves the small and the medium-sized fish.

A health worker must do the same thing as the fisherman if a patient has more than one psychiatric problem. Treat the biggest problem first, before treating medium-sized or small problems. If a patient has severe mental illness, depression and anxiety, treat the severe mental illness first. Severe mental illness is the patient's biggest problem. Depression is a medium-sized problem. Anxiety is the smallest problem.

Other symptoms that tell you a patient may have a psychiatric problem are:
• physical symptoms with no obvious cause
• tired all the time.

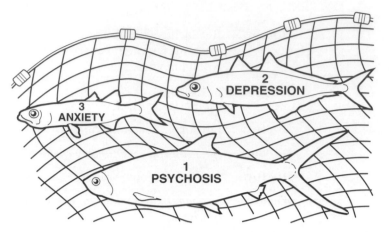

PICTURE 30 *Treat the most important psychiatric problem first*

Physical symptoms with no obvious cause

Some patients come to the health centre again and again with a physical symptom that has no obvious cause. Often the real problem is anxiety or depression. Ask the patient if there is anything which is making her worried or sad. Tell the patient that you think her symptoms are caused by worry or sadness. Counselling will often help these patients to find the reasons for their anxiety and to reduce their problems.

Tired all the time

Feeling tired all the time is very common in patients with psychiatric illnesses. If a patient tells you that he has been tired for a long time, he may have anaemia, diabetes or an infection. But, if there is no obvious physical cause for his tiredness, look for a psychiatric problem.

Refreshment break

Epilepsy

Epilepsy is usually caused by damage to part of the brain. It is not a psychiatric illness. However, many people *wrongly* think that people with epilepsy have a mental illness or that epilepsy is caused by spirits.

Patients with epilepsy have convulsions (also called fits). Convulsions can be caused by many other illnesses, such as very severe febrile diseases.

If a patient has had a convulsion:
- Treat him for a very severe febrile disease (see Chapter 2). If you know that he has epilepsy treat him for a very severe febrile disease only if he has more convulsions than usual *and* a fever. Send patients with a head injury to hospital if they have a convulsion.
- If there is no other illness that could have caused the convulsion, the patient may have epilepsy.

However, epilepsy is difficult to diagnose. If you think a patient may have epilepsy, you should send the patient to hospital for diagnosis. Doctors often only treat epilepsy patients with medicine if they have more than one convulsion every 2 months because epilepsy medicines can cause side effects, for example tiredness. The medicine prevents convulsions. Common medicines for epilepsy are phenobarbital, phenytoin and carbamazepine.

If a patient is taking epilepsy medicine, you need to:
- Explain to the patient and his family that epilepsy is caused by damage to the brain. This is especially important in cultures where people wrongly think that epilepsy is caused by evil spirits.
- Make sure the patient knows he must take the medicine every day. Tell the patient to get more medicine before the tablets finish.
- Tell the patient not to drive a car, lorry or motorcycle unless he has not had a convulsion for more than 3 years.

In areas with sleeping sickness

Tell your students:
Sleeping sickness is passed to people by the bite of some types of tsetse fly. Soon after the bite, the patient has an illness that is very similar to malaria. Later the brain becomes damaged. The most common symptom is sleeping during the day and not sleeping at night. The patient may develop severe mental illness and strange behaviour. The patient may find it difficult to walk. Patients with sleeping sickness will die without treatment. Send patients to hospital. Treatment is difficult.

SECTION 3: When to refer patients to hospital

Illnesses of the body may cause some psychiatric symptoms and need immediate treatment and referral to hospital.

POSTER 6:
(Student answer poster)

When to refer patients to hospital
Write the *headings and the left column only* of Table 1 on Poster 6.

Ask the students which patients with psychiatric symptoms or epilepsy need immediate hospital treatment. Ask what treatment they will give first.

TABLE 1 When to refer patients to hospital

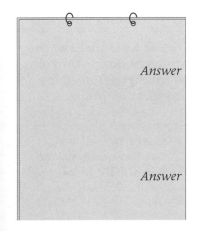

Symptom	Treatment and referral
Hallucinations or Delusions or Disorganised thoughts	If a patient has a **fever, treat for a very severe febrile disease** and send to hospital immediately. **If he has been hit on the head, send to hospital** immediately.
Alcohol withdrawal (very anxious, shaky or convulsion)	Give 10–20 mg **diazepam** and 50 ml of **milk or sugar water**. Send to hospital.

Answer

Answer

TABLE 1 *(continued)*

Symptom	Treatment and referral
Answer Epilepsy	**If** a patient with epilepsy has a **convulsion** for **more than 20 minutes** *or* has **more convulsions** than normal **and** has a **fever** *or* has a **general danger sign**, treat for very severe febrile disease and send to hospital immediately. If a patient with epilepsy has a **convulsion after a head injury**, send to hospital immediately.
Answer In areas with sleeping sickness: Sleeping during the day	**If** a patient **sleeps during** the **day**, but **not at night**, and **behaves strangely** or has **difficulty walking**, send to hospital immediately.

POSTER 7:
(Student answer poster)

When to refer patients to a psychiatric nurse or doctor

Write the *headings and the left column only* of Table 2 on Poster 7.

Ask the students to tell you which patients they would send to a psychiatric nurse or doctor.

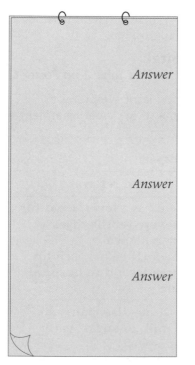

TABLE 2 When to refer patients to a psychiatric nurse or doctor

Symptom	Treatment and referral
Answer Acute dystonia	If you think that a patient has acute dystonia, treat with **trihexyphenidyl** (benzhexol). Send him to a psychiatric doctor or nurse immediately if you do not have any trihexyphenidyl (benzhexol).
Answer Depression	If a patient has **at least three of the** *extra* **symptoms of depression** or is **planning to kill herself**, send her to a psychiatric doctor or nurse immediately.
Answer Severe mental illness	If a patient has symptoms of severe mental illness but has **no fever** and has **not been hit on the head**, send him to see a psychiatric doctor or nurse immediately.

Section 4:   Practical: traditional healing

Ask the traditional healer to teach your students about his methods of treating anxiety and depression. Let him decide how to teach this section. Ask him to teach for about 30 minutes.

Section 5:   Answers to the quiz

Ask the students to call out the answers to each question in the quiz.

1. A patient is brought to you because he has been doing strange things for the past 5 days. What questions should you ask to find out if he has severe mental illness?
   - **When you are on your own, do you hear people's voices? Do you often see things that are unusual?**
   - **Do you have any ideas that other people know are not true that you know are true?**
   - **Have you been sad for more than 2 weeks?**

   Where should you send him if you think he has severe mental illness?
   - **If there is no fever and no head injury, send him to see a psychiatric doctor or nurse.**
   - **If there is fever, treat for a very severe febrile disease and send him to hospital immediately.**
   - **If he has had a head injury, send him to hospital immediately.**

2. What are the important symptoms of depression?
   - **Being very sad for at least 2 weeks**
   - **No interest in eating**
   - **Waking very early, well before sunrise**
   - **Being more sad in the morning than in the evening**
   - **Having no interest in sexual intercourse or other things that they normally enjoy**
   - **Being unable to concentrate or to do their work**
   - **Feeling no good or feeling bad for doing something wrong when they have not done anything wrong**
   - **Hoping to die or planning to kill himself**

3. What advice should you give to a patient who has epilepsy?
   - **Epilepsy is caused by damage in part of the brain. Epilepsy is not caused by evil spirits.**
   - **Do not drive for 3 years after a convulsion.**
   - **Take your epilepsy medicine every day and get more tablets before the tablets finish.**

Lesson 12 Tuberculosis and leprosy

BEFORE THE LESSON

- Arrange for all the students to visit a TB clinic and a leprosy clinic. It is best if all students visit the clinics before you teach this lesson. Ask the TB and leprosy doctors at the clinics to show the students each of the symptoms in the Table 1 in section 3.

- Give each student a copy of Table 1 'When to refer TB or leprosy patients to hospital' *before they visit the clinics*. They should take Table 1 with them when they visit the clinics.

- There are six posters in this lesson. (See p. 4 for information on how to use the posters.)
  Prepared posters 1, 3, 5, 6.
  Student answer posters: 2, 4.

SECTION 1:   Quiz

POSTER 1:
(Prepared poster)

Quiz

Ask the students to answer the questions on their own. Do not give the answers until the end of the lesson.

> 1. Name three important symptoms of tuberculosis (TB).
> 2. What investigations can be done to help decide if a patient has TB?
> 3. Name three important symptoms of leprosy.

SECTION 2:   Diagnosis and management

Tuberculosis

POSTER 2:
(Student answer poster)

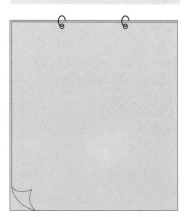

Tuberculosis

Divide Poster 2 into four areas. Label the four areas: Area 1: What is TB and who gets TB? Area 2: What symptoms does TB cause? Area 3: How is TB diagnosed in the clinic? and Area 4: TB treatment. In each of the four areas, write an example of a key word, for example:

Area 1: What is TB and who gets TB? **mycobacteria**	Area 2: What symptoms does TB cause? **cough for more than 3 weeks**
Area 3: How is TB diagnosed in the clinic? **sputum smear microscopy**	Area 4: TB treatment **treatment takes 6–8 months**

Ask each student to write one word or idea about TB in the correct area on Poster 2. Next, ask students to write other words or ideas on Poster 2.

Add any summary words from the information below that the students have missed.

Then, for each area in turn, ask each student to tell the class what he understands about the word he wrote. Draw a circle around each summary word as the student talks about it. Thank each student for his explanation.

Use the following explanations to add useful information and to correct mistakes.

Area 1: What is TB and who gets TB?

Tuberculosis (TB) is an illness that is caused by **mycobacteria**. Mycobacteria are like bacteria but multiply very slowly. Mycobacteria sometimes stop growing and hide in the body. This makes illnesses caused by mycobacteria difficult to treat.

TB mycobacteria cause abscesses. **TB abscesses** grow very slowly and are **not hot or red**. TB abscesses normally grow in the lungs. They also grow in lymph nodes, in joints, in bone or even in the brain.

When there are TB abscesses in the lungs, this is called pulmonary TB. When a TB abscess in a lung bursts, pus comes out and may get into the bronchi. Patients with pulmonary TB cough up this pus and spray TB mycobacteria into the air. Other people can **only get infected** with TB **by breathing in TB mycobacteria**. People who spend a lot of time in the same room as a patient with pulmonary TB are most likely to catch TB, especially if air cannot easily pass through the room.

When a person breathes in a large number of TB mycobacteria, the mycobacteria attack their body. If the person is healthy, their immune system (the body's defence system) will kill most of the mycobacteria. But a few of the TB mycobacteria will find a place to hide and go to sleep. The mycobacteria will wake up and attack the body again **if** the person's **immune system** is damaged or **weak**ened. For example, **HIV**, or **malnutrition** or **diabetes**, stop the immune system from fighting off illnesses such as TB. If the TB mycobacteria multiply, the **person will become ill with TB**.

Area 2: What symptoms does TB cause?

Most patients who are ill with tuberculosis have pulmonary tuberculosis. Patients with TB abscesses in the lymph nodes, joints, bones, abdomen, brain or area around the heart have extra-pulmonary TB. One in every five TB patients has extra-pulmonary TB.

(*continued*)

The most common symptoms of TB are:

1. **cough** for more than **3 weeks**
2. **lost weight** and does not have another illness which causes weight loss
3. **swelling of a lymph node** for more than **2 weeks** (The swelling is not hot and is not painful when touched.)
4. **coughing up blood**
5. **constant pain in the back** for more than 6 weeks and **part of** the **spine** is **tender.**

*Send a patient who has any of these symptoms to the TB clinic. Depending on where the TB abscesses are, TB (and other diseases) can cause **heart failure, septic arthritis, pain in the side of the chest,** or **strange behaviour**.*

Area 3: How TB is diagnosed in the clinic

Three tests can be used to help diagnose TB:

- **Sputum smear microscopy** is the most commonly used test. Three samples of a patient's sputum are examined under the microscope. If the patient has pulmonary TB, sputum smear microscopy may find **acid fast bacilli (AFB)**. TB mycobacteria are acid fast bacilli. Acid fast bacilli are often not found in the sputum of a patient with TB.
- **Chest X-ray** will show a shadow in the lung if the patient has a large TB abscess.
- **Tuberculin skin testing** is helpful for diagnosing TB in children. This is because children with TB do not usually produce sputum and chest X-rays in children do not always give clear results.

Area 4: TB treatment

TB mycobacteria can only be killed when they are multiplying. Because TB mycobacteria multiply very slowly, it takes several months to kill them all. The treatment for TB is different in different countries. Teach your students the treatment and drugs that are recommended by the national policy of your country. The treatment is also different if the patient has been treated for TB before.

Medicines used to treat TB are **rifampicin, isoniazid, pyrazinamide, streptomycin, ethambutol** or **thioacetazone**. Usually patients take three or four different medicines for the first 2 months of treatment. Next, patients take two medicines for a further 4–6 months.

Many countries now use **Directly Observed Treatment (DOT)** programmes. This means that patients are only treated in hospital until they can no longer infect other people. This is usually about 2 weeks. After this, patients can take their medicine at home. A reliable person in their community gives the patient the medicine. This person may be a shopkeeper, a village leader or a health worker in the village or at a hospital.

Side effects of TB medicines

TB medicines can cause side effects. Most of these side effects are mild and should not stop patients from taking the medicine.

However, sometimes TB medicines can make patients very ill:

- If a patient becomes **jaundiced**, stop the TB medicines and send the patient to the TB clinic.
- **Thioacetazone** can cause skin rash or blisters around the eyes or mouth. If the patient also has a fever, stop the TB medicines and send him to hospital immediately. If the patient does not have a fever, stop the thioacetazone and send him to the next TB clinic. Thioacetazone can have very bad side effects (called **Stevens–Johnson syndrome**) in patients who have HIV. If you know that a patient has HIV, do not give him thioacetazone.
- **Ethambutol** in large doses can cause **blindness**.

POSTER 3:
(Prepared poster)

What to tell TB patients

What to tell TB patients:
- The **treatment will take 6–8 months**.
- He **cannot** infect other people **2 weeks after** starting the **treatment**.
- If he **does not complete** the **treatment**, he **will become ill with TB again**. After **incomplete treatment** the TB mycobacteria are **more dangerous** to him and to other people.
- He should **exercise** if he feels well enough.
- **Streptomycin** is dangerous to unborn babies. If a woman could become pregnant, she must tell the TB clinic immediately.
- Other TB treatments are safe for pregnant women.
- Rifampicin makes sweat, tears, **urine and semen red or orange** in colour. The semen is healthy and **men may safely father children** when they are taking TB treatment.
- The patient can have **sexual intercourse**.
- If the white parts of the **eyes become yellow**, the patient should **stop the medicine** and **go to** the **TB clinic**.
- If the patient is taking **thioacetazone** and develops a **rash or blisters around his eyes**, he should **stop the medicine** and **go to** the **TB clinic**.

Refreshment break

Leprosy

POSTER 4:
(Student answer poster)

Leprosy

Divide Poster 4 into four areas. Label the four areas: Area 1: What is leprosy? Who gets leprosy?, Area 2: Leprosy symptoms,

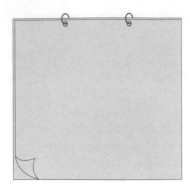

Area 3: Diagnosing leprosy in the clinic, Area 4: Leprosy treatment. This is Poster 4.

Ask each student to write one word or idea about leprosy in the correct area on Poster 4. Next, ask students to write other words or ideas on Poster 4. Add any summary words from the information below that the students have missed. Then, for each area in turn, ask each student to tell the class what she understands about the word she wrote. Draw a circle around each word as the student talks about it. Thank each student for her explanation.

Use the following explanations to add useful information and to correct mistakes.

Area 1: What is leprosy and who gets leprosy?

Leprosy is caused by *Mycobacterium leprae*. These mycobacteria grow on the **cold parts of the body**, for example on the **face** and **buttocks, inside** the **nose** and **in the nerves under the skin**. Like TB mycobacteria, leprosy mycobacteria grow very slowly. This is why you will rarely see young children with leprosy. When a patient with leprosy mycobacteria in the nose coughs or sneezes, the mycobacteria are sprayed into the air and may be **breathed in** by other people. Most people are able to kill all of the leprosy mycobacteria that they breathe in. People who are less able to fight off leprosy mycobacteria will become ill with leprosy after a few years. People with HIV infection are *not* more likely than other people to become ill with leprosy.

The type of leprosy a person gets depends on how many of the leprosy mycobacteria his body can kill:

- If only a few of the mycobacteria are killed, the patient will develop **lepromatous leprosy**.
- If some of mycobacteria are killed, the patient will develop **borderline leprosy**.
- If most of the mycobacteria are killed, the patient will develop **tuberculoid leprosy**.

Another name for leprosy is Hansen's disease.

Area 2: What symptoms does leprosy cause?

Leprosy causes symptoms in the places where the leprosy mycobacteria grow:

- If leprosy grows in the skin, it makes the **skin go pale** (in dark-skinned people) **or red** (in light-skinned people). Leprosy can also cause loss of feeling in the skin.
- If leprosy grows in a nerve, it will damage the nerve. This can **stop** the **muscles** from **working** and the patient may not be able to move part of his body. It can also **stop** the patient from **feeling** things. If he cannot feel hot or sharp things he may damage himself.

(*continued*)
- Patients who have lepromatous leprosy and borderline leprosy may have corneal ulceration and **poor eyesight**.

Send a patient with any of these symptoms to the leprosy clinic:

1. An area of the **skin** has become **pale** or red. Ask the patient to close his eyes. Touch the pale area with the corner of a piece of cloth. If the patient is **not able to feel** the cloth, send him to the leprosy clinic.
2. A pale area of skin is **no better after** using a **treatment for fungus infection** for 4 weeks.
3. An **unusual feeling** in an arm, leg or on the face.
4. **Painless ulcers or burns** on his feet or hands.
5. **Swelling in the skin**, often in the ears, which is not painful. The swollen skin does not sweat and loses hair. It is common for people with leprosy to lose the outer part of the eyebrows.
6. A **nerve is painful when you touch it**. Common places to find painful nerves are in the neck, above the elbows, at the wrists, the side of the knees and at the ankles. The nerves feel like dead worms when you touch them.

If a patient cannot feel a corner of cloth touching her feet, she may have leprosy. Patients with anaemia, malnutrition or tiredness may also tell you that they cannot feel their feet but they can feel cloth touching their feet.

Area 3: How leprosy is diagnosed in the clinic
Leprosy is usually diagnosed by just **examining the patient.** Sometimes **skin-slit smear** microscopy is needed. The doctor makes small cuts in several parts of the patient's skin and takes scrapes of the patient's skin to look at under a microscope. Microscopy of smears of this skin may find acid fast bacilli (AFB). Leprosy mycobacteria are acid fast bacilli.

Area 4: Leprosy treatment
Leprosy mycobacteria multiply very slowly, so it takes several months to kill all of them. Medicines used to treat leprosy are **dapsone, rifampicin** and **clofazimine.**
- **Tuberculoid leprosy** – Patients are **treated for 6 months**, with dapsone 100 mg every day. They also take rifampicin 600 mg once a month, usually in the clinic. Patients continue to be **seen in** the **leprosy clinic for 2 years**.
- **Borderline and lepromatous leprosy** – Patients with borderline or lepromatous leprosy are **treated for 24 months**. They take dapsone 100 mg and clofazimine 50 mg every day. Patients also take rifampicin 600 mg and clofazimine 300 mg once each month, usually in the clinic. Patients **go to** the **leprosy clinic for 5 years**.

Side effects of leprosy medicines

Dapsone sometimes makes the patient very ill 4–6 weeks after starting treatment. Stop the medicine and send the patient to hospital immediately. Patients usually have damaged nerves by the time treatment for leprosy is started. Treatment often damages nerves causing lack of feeling or weakness in a part of the body.

POSTER 5:
(Prepared poster)

Advice for patients with leprosy

- She **cannot infect** other people **3 days after** starting the **treatment.**
- **If** she **does not complete** the **treatments** she **will become ill again**. Leprosy mycobacteria are **more difficult to treat after incomplete treatment.**
- She can **exercise** if she feels well enough.
- Leprosy medicines are dangerous to unborn babies. Women should **not** get **pregnant** while taking leprosy medicines.
- Rifampicin and clofazimine make sweat, tears, **urine and semen red or orange** in colour. The semen is healthy and **men may safely father children** when taking leprosy medicines. Leprosy is not passed on to children.
- Patients can have **sexual intercourse**. Leprosy is not passed on during sexual intercourse.
- If you become very ill 4–6 weeks after starting dapsone treatment, stop the medicine and go to hospital immediately.

For patients taking clofazimine:
- Clofazimine may cause the **skin** to become **orange** or purple and the skin of the arms and legs to become dry.
- Clofazimine may also cause **abdominal pains** or **diarrhoea**. Do not stop the medicine.

Patients with tuberculoid leprosy:
- Treatment takes 6 months.

Patients with borderline leprosy:
- Treatment takes 2 years.
- Part of the body may become very **painful** and **swollen** or **weak**. This is a called a **reversal reaction**. Do not stop the medicine. **Take paracetamol**, two tablets four times a day. Go to the leprosy clinic.

Patients with lepromatous leprosy:
- Treatment takes 2 years.
- The patient may have a **fever** that does not get better after treatment for malaria. This is called an ENL reaction. Do not stop the leprosy medicine. Take **paracetamol**, two tablets four times a day, and go to the leprosy clinic.

Nerve damage means that many leprosy patients cannot feel parts of their feet or hands. Advise patients to give their feet and hands special treatment every day to prevent the skin becoming broken and ulcerated.

POSTER 6:
(Prepared poster)

Skin treatment advice

- **Look at** your **feet, hands** and **eyes every day**. Use a mirror or ask a friend to look at your eyes.
- **Soak** your **feet in water mixed with vegetable oil**. Coconut oil is suitable.
- **Remove hard skin** by rubbing gently with a rough stone.
- Put **vegetable oil or petroleum jelly** on your hands and feet.
- **Clean and cover wounds**.
- Every day **stretch** the parts of your body that you cannot use.
- Protect your hands with **gloves** or a cloth when you cook or work.
- Protect your feet with **shoes**. These must be the correct size, have a soft rubber sole and be soft inside.
- Wear **sunglasses** during the day. **Cover** your **eyes with** a **cloth at night**. Your doctor may give you eye drops to stop your eyes from becoming dry.

SECTION 3: When to refer patients to hospital

Before the lesson, give each student a copy of Table 1, which explains when to send patients to a clinic or hospital. They should take this table with them when they visit the TB and leprosy clinics.

TABLE 1 When to refer TB and leprosy patients to hospital

TB PATIENTS

Refer to TB clinic for diagnosis if:
- cough more than 3 weeks
- weight loss
- lymph node swollen for more than 2 weeks
- coughing up blood
- pain in back for more than 6 weeks and part of the spine feels tender

Stop TB medicine and send to the TB clinic if:
- jaundice
- rash or blisters

(continued)

LEPROSY PATIENTS
Refer to the leprosy clinic for diagnosis if:
- pale or red skin areas and no feeling in the skin
- strange feeling in arm, leg or face
- ulcers or burns, which are not painful
- painful nerves

Send to hospital immediately if:
- using dapsone and has fever and rash – stop dapsone

Continue leprosy medicines, give paracetamol and send to the leprosy clinic if:
- borderline leprosy with painful skin or weak foot or hand
- lepromatous leprosy with fever, if no better after first-line malaria treatment

SECTION 4: Practical: Visits to a TB clinic and a leprosy clinic

Each student should visit a TB clinic and a leprosy clinic during the course.

SECTION 5: Answers to the quiz

Ask the students to call out the answers to each question in the quiz.

1. Name three important symptoms of TB.
   - **A cough for more than 3 weeks**
   - **Weight loss**
   - **Swelling of a lymph node for more than 2 weeks**
   - **Coughing up blood**
   - **A constant pain in the back for more than 6 weeks and part of the spine is tender**

2. What investigations can be done in the clinic to diagnose TB?
   - **Sputum smear microscopy**
   - **Chest X-ray**
   - **Tuberculin testing**

3. Name three important symptoms of leprosy.
   - **Pale skin with loss of feeling**
   - **Ulcers or burns on the hands or feet which are not painful**
   - **Swelling in the skin which is not painful**
   - **Pain on touching a nerve**

Lesson 13   HIV disease

BEFORE THE LESSON

■ There are seven posters in this lesson. (See p. 4 for information on how to use the posters.)
Prepared poster: 1
Student answer posters: 2, 3, 4, 5, 7. Only write the title on Poster 5 – the students will complete Poster 5 during the lesson.
Summary poster: 6

■ Prepare one copy of Table 1 in section 3 for each student.

■ For the practical in section 4, you will need:
   – one white cup for each student
   – enough water to fill each cup one-third full
   – enough starch solution to fill *one* or *two* cups one-third full
   – an instruction card for each student, prepared before the lesson
   – 10 ml of polyvidone iodine 10%. Keep this separate.

| How to prepare the instruction cards | For the practical, give each student one of four different types of cards. The instruction cards will tell students with whom they should mix their water. |

1. One or two cards should say:
'You sleep with anyone. Mix your water with 10 or more other people's water.' (If you have 20 students, make one card with these instructions. If you have more than 20 students, make two cards.)

2. Half of the cards should say:
'You sleep with 4 or 5 people. You do not use condoms. Mix your water with 4 or 5 different people's water.'
(So, if you have 20 students, make 10 cards with these instructions.)

Divide the remaining cards into two more or less equal groups:

3. Some cards say:
'You only sleep with one other person. Mix your water with *one other person's* water. Do this *with the same person* 4 times.'
(So, if you have 20 students, make four cards with these instructions.)

4. Some cards say:
'You sleep with two or three people. You always use condoms. *Talk* to two or three other people. *Do not mix your water with anyone.*'
(So, if you have 20 students, make four cards with these instructions.)

Preparation on the morning of the lesson

1. Make the starch solution by mixing mix ½ teaspoon of clothes starch (or maize flour or cassava flour) in a cup which is one-third full of water (or water that has been used to cook rice). *If you use flour instead of starch, or rice water instead of water, test that the game will work before the lesson.*

2. In the classroom: fill *one cup only* one-third full with starch solution. If you have more than 20 students, fill 2 cups one-third with starch solution. Fill *all other cups* one-third full with *water. Make sure that you do this before the students arrive.*

SECTION 1:   Quiz

POSTER 1:
(Prepared poster)

Quiz
Ask the students to answer the questions on their own. Do not give the answers until the end of the lesson.

1. How is HIV passed from one person to another?
2. Which illnesses does HIV make more common?
3. If a patient is infected with HIV today, when will a blood test show that he has been infected with HIV?
4. How can we prevent people from becoming infected with HIV?

SECTION 2:   Diagnosis and management

POSTER 2:
(Student answer poster)

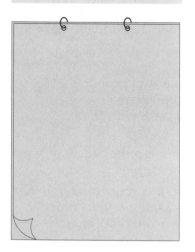

HIV and AIDS
Divide Poster 2 into four areas. Label the four areas: Area 1: What are HIV and AIDS? How are they transmitted?; Area 2: What illnesses are made more common by HIV?; Area 3: How to diagnose HIV in the clinic; Area 4: Treatment for HIV disease and how to prevent HIV infections.
Ask each student to write one word or idea about HIV and AIDS in the correct area on Poster 2. Next, ask students to write other words or ideas on Poster 2. Add any summary words from the information below that the students have missed. Then, for each of the four areas in turn, ask each student to tell the class what she understands about the word she wrote. Draw a circle around each summary word as the student talks about it. Thank each student for her explanation.
Use the following explanations to add useful information and to correct mistakes.

Area 1: What are HIV and AIDS and how are they transmitted?
The Human Immunodeficiency Virus (HIV) slowly **kills** the body's **white blood cells**. The white cells help to protect the body against infections. Many people with HIV

(*continued*)

infection have no symptoms and stay well for months or years. As HIV kills more and more white blood cells, the patient will get more common infections. These common infections kill many patients in poor and tropical countries. If a person who has HIV infection lives for several years, he will become ill with **unusual diseases**. When this happens, the patient has **Acquired Immunodeficiency Syndrome** (**AIDS**). Many patients with HIV infection **have no symptoms** and are well. Other HIV patients have many swellings in the neck and under the arms. These swellings are smaller than 6 cm across.

HIV is **passed** from one **person to** other **persons**:

- during sexual intercourse **if** a **condom** is **not used** (**Other sexually transmitted diseases** also help HIV to infect other people.)
- **by blood transfusion** if blood is not tested for HIV
- by using **needles** that have **not** been **sterilised** for injecting medicines or drugs
- **from** an **HIV-infected mother to her baby**, during **pregnancy, birth** or through **breastfeeding**. About one of every three babies born to mothers who have HIV are infected with HIV.

Tell your students:

There is a risk that a mother who has HIV can pass on HIV if she breastfeeds her baby. However, even for mothers who have HIV, breastfeeding their baby is usually safer than bottle feeding. Bottle feeding with artificial feeds, like baby formula (substitutes for breast milk), can be dangerous. If a mother bottlefeeds her child, the risk of the child dying from other illnesses, like malnutrition, pneumonia or diarrhoea, is increased 25 times.

*If a mother has HIV, it is **only** safer to use artificial feeds instead of breastfeeding **if** the mother is able to sterilise the bottles and buy enough baby formula to mix it correctly with safe, clean water **at all times**.*

HIV is **not transmitted**:
- by **mosquito bites**
- by **sharing food, tools for eating** or by **touching unbroken skin**.

Area 2: Illnesses which are made more common by HIV
People with HIV are more likely to get some infections and illnesses. The following illnesses are made more common by HIV:

1. **herpes zoster**
2. **pneumonia**, *Pneumocystis carinii* **pneumonia (PCP), sinusitis**
3. **tuberculosis**

4. oral candida
5. oral hairy leucoplakia
6. **weight loss, persistent diarrhoea**
7. **parotitis**
8. **non-typhi salmonellae**
9. **Kaposi's sarcoma**
10. **cryptococcus.**

If a patient has one of these illnesses, treat the illness and talk to the patient about HIV. If the patient is worried about HIV or thinks she may be infected, refer her to a voluntary counselling and testing centre.

Area 3: How HIV is diagnosed in the clinic
HIV is usually diagnosed with a test called an **antibody test**. The test looks for antibodies to the virus in a sample of the patient's blood. The body's immune system produces antibodies to HIV after infection with the virus. It can take up to 8 weeks for the body to produce antibodies. An **HIV test** will **not show whether** a **patient** has been **infected** with HIV **until up to 8 weeks after the infection**.

Area 4: Treatment for HIV and AIDS
There is **no treatment** available that **can completely cure HIV**. But:

- People with HIV can be **treated for other infections**.
- Children and adults can have all the usual **immunisations**.
- **Pregnant women** can **take vitamin A** in the last 3 months of pregnancy to reduce the chance of passing HIV to their babies.
- People with HIV can cope better with their illness if they receive **counselling** and practical help.
- You can help people with HIV to **stay well** by advising them to eat a **mixed diet**, including five pieces of fruit or vegetables every day, and to **go for treatment quickly** if they get ill.

Treatment for infections and illnesses which are made more common by HIV

POSTER 3:
(Student answer poster)

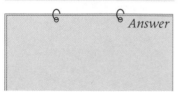

How to treat illnesses made more common by HIV
Ask the students how to treat the infections and illnesses below.

1. **Herpes zoster (shingles)** – Herpes zoster causes an area of skin on one side of the body to become red, blistered, ulcerated and painful. **Treat** in the **same** way **as** any **ulcer. Clean and cover the skin**. When the ulceration heals, it normally leaves a scar.

Answer

2. **Pneumonia or sinusitis** – If the patient has had pneumonia or sinusitis two times or more this year, he may have HIV infection. See Lesson 2.
   PCP. PCP is a type of pneumonia. PCP is short for *Pneumocystis carinii* **pneumonia**. If a **child less than one year old has a cough for more than 3 weeks**, he may have PCP. Send him to hospital.
   Sinusitis is an infection of a sinus. If a patient has pain in the face and yellow or green discharge coming from his nose, diagnose sinusitis. **Treat** with **antibiotics for 10 days**. Give children aged 12 or less amoxicillin or co-trimoxazole. Give patients aged 13 and over who are not pregnant, tetracycline 250 mg four times a day.

Answer

3. **Tuberculosis** – see Lesson 12.

Answer

4. **Oral candida** – Oral candida (sometimes called thrush) causes a painful mouth. See Lesson 14.

Answer

5. **Oral hairy leucoplakia** – You will find white lines on the side of the tongue. Oral hairy leukoplakia is painless and **needs no treatment**.

Answer

6. **Weight loss with persistent diarrhoea** – Patients with HIV may have diarrhoea and fever often. This causes weight loss. Sometimes the diarrhoea is caused by unusual parasites. If the patient is dehydrated **give oral rehydration solution** (see Lesson 6). If he is not dehydrated, advise him to drink plenty of fluids. Advise all patients to eat a **mixed diet**. Send to hospital.

Answer

7. **Parotitis** – If a child **between 1 year old and 2 years old** has a painful swelling over the angle of the jaw, the child has **parotitis** and may have HIV. (Mumps can also cause parotitis and a fever. Mumps usually affects children aged over 5 years.) Give **paracetamol for pain** if needed.

Show students where the angle of the jaw is.

Patients with more advanced HIV disease or AIDS may get other illnesses, including non-typhi salmonellae, Kaposi's sarcoma and cryptococcus.

Answer

- **Non-typhi salmonellae** in HIV patients is like typhoid. Patients have fever that does not get better with malaria treatment, and they need to go **to hospital**.

Answer

- **Kaposi's sarcoma** is a cancer which shows as purple patches on the body. It grows slowly and usually **does not need treatment**.

Answer

- **Cryptococcus** is an infection that can cause a constant headache. It cannot usually be cured. You can give the patient **ibuprofen** 400 mg three times a day to reduce the pain.

How to prevent HIV infections

POSTER 4:
(Student answer poster)

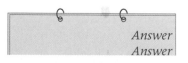

Answer

Answer

Answer

Answer

Answer

Answer

Answer

How to prevent HIV infections
Ask the students how to prevent HIV infections.

1. Teach people to **use condoms** during sexual intercourse. Condoms protect against HIV and other sexually transmitted diseases.

2. Send people for **treatment for other sexually transmitted diseases**, and ask them to take their partners for treatment (see Poster 5).

3. Make sure **blood for transfusion is safe** by testing it for HIV. Reduce unnecessary blood transfusions. Only give blood if it is needed to save a patient's life. Only give a transfusion:
   - if a patient has a haemoglobin (Hb) of 5 g/dl or less
   - if a woman in the last month of pregnancy has haemoglobin of 7 g/dl or less
   - if a patient is bleeding very heavily and the bleeding is not stopping.

4. Use **safe procedures in health centres**:
   - cover open wounds or cuts on your hands and arms
   - make sure that needles and syringes are properly sterilised
   - put used needles in a tin with a lid to avoid injuries. Bury the tin if you do not re-use and sterilise the needles.

   If a health worker cuts her skin with a dirty needle, she should make the cut bleed for 2 minutes. Next, wash the cut with soap and water. Some countries have medicines which can be used immediately to reduce the chance of injured health workers becoming infected with HIV.

5. **Counsel pregnant women** about HIV testing if it is possible to feed babies safely without breastfeeding.

6. Counsel pregnant women about HIV testing if special treatments are available to help prevent the baby from getting HIV from its mother during pregnancy and birth.

7. Teach people who inject drugs how to **sterilise needles and syringes** with bleach and water.

Sexually transmitted diseases

POSTER 5:
(Student answer poster)

Answer
Answer

Symptoms of sexually transmitted diseases
Ask the students to tell you the symptoms of sexually transmitted diseases (STDs).

1. **ulcers** on or near the private parts
2. passing **pus** or unusual material from the private parts

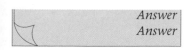

Answer
Answer

3. **pain** on **passing urine**
4. **pain on** having **sexual intercourse**

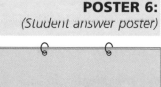

POSTER 6:
(Student answer poster)

Who needs to know about HIV and AIDS?

Ask your students which people need to know how to prevent HIV. Summarise their ideas on Poster 6 as students call them out. After the students have finished giving you their ideas, tell them *that all answers to this question are correct*. It is important for *everyone* to know about HIV and AIDS. *Everyone* needs to know how to prevent HIV infections.

Answer

Use a thick pen or large letters to write '**Everyone**' on Poster 6.

Refreshment break

How to counsel people about an HIV test

Counselling means helping patients to decide what to do. Your job is to answer questions and give the patient information so that he can decide what he wants to do. It is not your job to tell the patient what to do. Only the patient can decide whether he wants to have an HIV test.

POSTER 7:
(Summary poster)

How to counsel patients about HIV testing

1. Tell the patient (or the mother if the patient is a child) **why you think** that **he may have HIV**.

2. Explain to the patient that there is **no treatment that will remove HIV**. Explain that there are **treatments for** the **infections which are made more common by HIV**.

3. **Give** the patient **time to understand** what you have said to him.

4. **Encourage the patient to ask questions**. Answer questions and make sure the patient understands the information.

5. Talk to the patient about what may happen if he knows that he has HIV. If he knows that he is infected with HIV, he will be able to plan what to do with the rest of his life. Let the patient decide whether he wants to be tested for HIV.

6. Talk to the patient about what may happen if other people know he has HIV. Telling a close friend or relative can help the patient to cope. But it can also cause problems. For example, a woman may fear that her husband will leave her or that her family will reject her. It can be helpful for **all members of a family** to have counselling before someone is tested for HIV. Let the patient decide whether he wants the family to have counselling with him.

7. **Teach** the patient **how to prevent** other people from becoming infected with **HIV**.

SECTION 3: When to refer patients

Give each of your students a copy of Table 1.

TABLE 1 When to refer patients who may have HIV to hospital

Refer urgently to hospital or clinic for diagnosis and treatment if:
- The patient's fever is no better 2 days after treatment for malaria.
- The patient is a child less than 1 year old who has had a cough for more than 3 weeks.
- The patient has a severe headache and difficulty moving their neck or is behaving strangely.

Refer to the next clinic for diagnosis and treatment if:
- The patient has a sexually transmitted disease (send to the STD clinic).
- The patient has had a cough for more than 3 weeks or has blood in the sputum (send to the TB clinic).
- The patient has lost weight with no obvious cause.
- The patient has had diarrhoea for more than 2 weeks.
- The patient has severe herpes zoster.
- The patient has unusual skin rashes, especially if the patient is using thioacetazone. Stop the thioacetazone.

Refer for counselling and testing if:
- A patient wants to know if they have been infected with HIV.
- The patient has had herpes zoster, or oral candida or oral hairy leucoplakia.
- The patient has Kaposi's sarcoma.
- A child aged between 1 and 2 years has parotitis.
- A patient has had sinusitis or pneumonia two or more times in one year.

SECTION 4: Practical: How to avoid HIV

Tell your students that this game shows how easy it is for HIV to infect a large number of people. Make sure your students understand that in this game, they are *only pretending* to have sexual intercourse and they are *only pretending* to pass on HIV infection.

Some students may find a game about sexual intercourse embarrassing. Tell your students that HIV is a very important and serious health problem. This game will help them to understand how HIV is passed from one person to another person and they will be able to advise their patients better.

Game

Give a cup and an instruction card to each student (see page 169). Give one student the cup with starch solution and a card with the instruction 'You sleep with anyone...'. Give all other students cups with water and a card.

Do not tell this student or the other students that one cup is different from the other cups. It is important that none of the students knows that one cup is different. This cup is the source of the 'HIV infection' in the game.

Tell the students:

- In this game, the water in the cups represents body fluids. Each time you mix your water with someone else's water, this represents sexual intercourse.
- Your card tells you who you can mix your water with. Follow the instructions on your card. Remember that if your card says 'You always use condoms', you *must not* mix your water with anyone else's water.
- You have 10 to 15 minutes to play the game. Walk around the classroom and talk to at least four other students. Tell each student you talk to what is written on your card.
- If your card *and* the card of the student you are talking to tells you to mix water together, pour *all* your water into the other person's cup. Next, pour *half* of the water back into your own cup.

After 10 to 15 minutes:

- Tell the students that you will test the water. You will pretend to test their 'blood' for HIV.
- Tell the students that the water in their cup will turn blue or black if they have 'been infected with HIV' during the game. Tell them the water will turn yellow or brown if they have 'not been infected with HIV'.
- Put four drops of polyvidone iodine 10% into each cup. Show the students that some of the water has turned blue or black and that some of the water has turned yellow or brown.
- Tell the students that at the beginning of the game, only one person in the class was 'infected with HIV'.
- Ask if anyone knew who was infected before the game. *Do not tell the students who was infected.*
- Tell the students what was written on the cards of the students who 'were infected with HIV' during the game.
- Next, tell the students what was written on the cards of the students who were 'not infected with HIV' during the game.
- Ask the students what they have learnt from this game. Look for the following answers:

Answer   Most people with HIV do not know that they are infected. They may infect a large number of other people without knowing.

Answer   It is not possible to know from looking at a person if he is infected with HIV or not.

Answer   Condoms protect against HIV infection.

Answer   If a person only has one sexual partner, he may still become infected with HIV if his partner has other sexual partners.

Answer   People who have many sexual partners and who do not use condoms are most likely to become infected with HIV.

This is why it is important to teach everyone about HIV infection and to advise people to use condoms every time they have sexual intercourse.

SECTION 5:   Answers to the quiz
Ask the students to call out the answers to each question in the quiz.

1. How is HIV passed from one person to another?
   - **Unprotected sexual intercourse (without a condom)**
   - **Infected blood transfusion**
   - **Unsterilised needles and syringes used for injecting medicines or drugs**
   - **From an infected mother to her baby during pregnancy, birth or through breastfeeding**

2. What infections and illnesses does HIV make more common?

   - **Herpes zoster**
   - **Pneumonia**
   - **Tuberculosis**
   - **Oral candida**
   - **Oral hairy leucoplakia**

   - **Diarrhoea**
   - **Parotitis**
   - **Non-typhi salmonella**
   - **Cryptococcus**
   - **Kaposi's sarcoma**

3. If a patient is infected with HIV today, when will a blood test show that he has been infected with HIV?
   - **Up to 8 weeks after the infection**

4. How can we prevent people from becoming infected with HIV?
   - **Encourage people to use condoms during sexual intercourse.**
   - **Send people for treatment for other sexually transmitted diseases and ask them to take their partners for treatment.**
   - **Make sure blood for transfusion is safe by testing it for HIV. Only give blood if it is needed to save a patient's life.**
   - **Using safe procedures in health centres.**
   - **Teach people who inject drugs how to sterilise needles and syringes with bleach and water.**

Ear, nose and throat problems

BEFORE THE LESSON

- There are five posters in this lesson. (See p. 4 for information on how to use the posters.)
  Prepared posters: 1, 2, 3
  Summary posters: 4, 5

- Give each student a copy of Appendix 20.

- Ask one student to teach the other students how to make a toothbrush in section 2. He will need a piece of soft wood (for example, from a banana tree) and a knife.

- Prepare one copy of Tables 1 to 4 in section 3 for each student.

- You need a syringe (5 ml or larger), a cup of water, some soap, a bowl and a towel or cloth for the practical in section 4.

SECTION 1: Quiz

POSTER 1:
(Prepared poster)

Quiz

Ask the students to answer the questions on their own. Do not give the answers until the end of the lesson.

1. A patient has a fever and a yellow or green discharge from his ear. How will you treat him?
2. What are the symptoms of diphtheria? How do you treat diphtheria?
3. What are the symptoms of epiglottitis? How do you treat epiglottitis?

SECTION 2: Diagnosis and management

Today you will learn about the most common and important ear, nose and throat problems. It is unusual for these problems to cause death.
If a patient has a problem that you do not know how to treat, send him to the ear, nose and throat clinic.

Ear problems

Ask the students to look at Appendix 20 and to tell you what the common symptoms of ear problems are.

Pain or swelling

If a patient has **pain in the ear or swelling near the ear**, press behind the outside part of the ear, the ear hole and in front of the ear:

- If a patient has a **tender swelling behind the ear** she may have a bacterial infection called **mastoiditis**.
- If the **ear itself is swollen**, the patient may have a bacterial infection called **cellulitis**. Treat cellulitis or mastoiditis with an intramuscular injection of procaine penicillin fortified or chloramphenicol (not if pregnant, breastfeeding or less than 1 month old) or benzylpenicillin. Next, send the patient to hospital immediately.
- If a patient has a **tender ear hole**, she may have **infected otitis externa**. Treat infected otitis externa with co-trimoxazole and steroid ear drops for 5 days.
- If the area in front of the ear is tender and swollen, ask the patient to bite her teeth together. If the patient has a **tooth abscess**, it will be painful to bite her teeth together.
- If there is a **swelling in front of and below the ear**, the patient usually has **mumps**. Mumps is a virus infection which causes the parotid glands at the corner of the jaw to swell. Many patients with mumps have a swelling on both sides of the face. The patient does not need an antibiotic. Advise her to eat a mixed diet. Tell the patient that the swelling will go away after about 1 or 2 weeks.

Discharge

- If there is a **green or yellow discharge** from an ear, the patient may have **otitis media, infected otitis externa or a foreign body in the ear**. Treat with co-trimoxazole for 5 days in malaria areas. Or treat with amoxicillin if the patient is pregnant or there is no malaria in your area. If the discharge is no better 1 week after starting treatment, send the patient to the ear, nose and throat clinic.

Itching

- If there is itching in both ears, the patient may have **otitis externa**. Give steroid ear drops. Prednisolone, betamethasone or triamcinolone ear drops are all suitable. Give 2 drops three times a day for 5 days.

Noises in the ears

If the patient has **noises in the ears** (tinnitus) this may be caused by anaemia, fever or poor hearing.

- If the noise is in time with the heart beat, the tinnitus is usually caused by anaemia or fever. Anaemia and fever make the blood go through the ears faster than normal.
- If the noise is constant and not in time with the heart beat, the tinnitus is caused by poor hearing from wax blocking the ear.

Throat pain

If a patient has pain in his throat, take a history and look at the back of the throat. Do not put anything into the throat. If the

patient is a young child, the best time to look at the throat is
when he is crying.

Ask an older patient to:
- look towards the window
- look upwards a little
- open his mouth and say 'gaaaaaaaaa'.

POSTER 2:
(Prepared poster)

The throat
Draw Picture 31 on Poster 2.

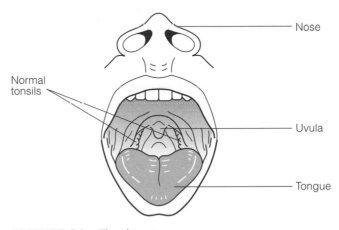

PICTURE 31   *The throat*

Show Poster 2 to the students and explain that:

Pain in the throat can be caused by tonsillitis, diphtheria or
epiglottitis.
- **Tonsillitis** is an infection of the tonsils. Tonsillitis is caused by a
  virus or bacteria. It is difficult to know which type of tonsillitis a
  patient has. Normal tonsils are often big and often have white
  areas in the cracks.
- **Epiglottitis** is an infection of the epiglottis. The epiglottis is a
  piece of gristle behind the tongue, which prevents food and
  drink from going into the lungs. Severe epiglottitis stops air from
  going into the lungs.
- **Diphtheria** is an infection caused by diphtheria bacteria.
  Diphtheria can damage the heart and nerves.

Diagnosis

POSTER 3:
(Prepared poster)

Causes of throat pain
Draw Pictures 32, 33 and 34 on Poster 3.
Explain Poster 3 to the students. Explain how to make a
diagnosis in a patient with a painful throat.

If the patient has a painful throat:
- and is **not able to drink**, diagnose **epiglottitis**
- and the throat is more **red** than usual but there are **no areas of
  white** on the tonsils, diagnose **tonsillitis caused by a virus**

181

- and the throat is **very red** and there are areas of **white only in** the **cracks of** the **tonsils**, diagnose **tonsillitis caused by bacteria**
- and there are **white or grey areas** which **cover the tonsils** but the throat is only **slightly red**, diagnose **diphtheria**.

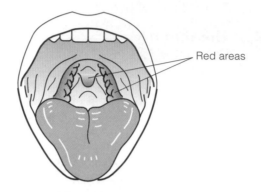

PICTURE 32 *Tonsillitis caused by a virus*

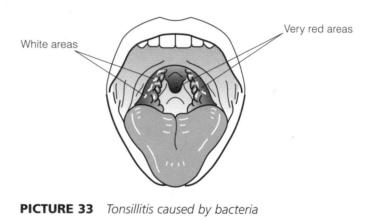

PICTURE 33 *Tonsillitis caused by bacteria*

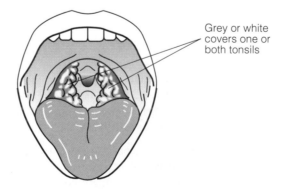

PICTURE 34 *Diphtheria in the throat*

How to treat patients with throat pain

POSTER 4:
(Summary poster)

How to treat throat problems

Summarise the treatment for each throat problem below on Poster 4 as you teach.

Tonsillitis caused by a virus

Husseini is 6 years old. He has had a painful throat and a fever for 2 days. He also has a cough and a fever. He is able to drink, is not anaemic and does not have fast breathing. Ask Husseini to look towards the window, look up a little and to open his mouth and say 'gaaaaa'. Husseini's throat is more red than usual. There are no areas of white on the tonsils, but the tonsils look very big. Husseini has tonsillitis caused by a virus.

Treatment: Tell Husseini's mother to **feed** him **five times a day** until 1 week after he is better. Give Husseini the first-line **malaria treatment**. Ask his mother to **bring** Husseini **back** to the health centre **if** he is **no better after 3 days**.

Tonsillitis caused by bacteria

Juma is an 8-year-old boy with fever and pain in his throat. His throat is very red. There are white areas in the cracks of his tonsils. Juma is able to drink. Juma has tonsillitis caused by a bacteria infection.

Treatment: Give Juma **phenoxymethylpenicillin** 250 mg three times a day for 5 days. (He weighs more than 20 kg but less than 40 kg.) Ask Juma's mother to bring him **back after 3 days if** he is **no better**. If there is malaria in your area you also give Juma the first-line malaria treatment if he is no better after 3 days.

Diphtheria

Amina is a 2-year-old girl who is unwell and has a painful throat. Amina was not given her immunisations. Amina has a fever but she is not anaemic and she does not have fast breathing. You look inside Amina's mouth when she coughs or cries. You can see large areas of **white or grey** on her throat. The white **areas cover both tonsils**. The throat is only **slightly red**. Amina's mouth smells bad. Amina has diphtheria.

Treatment: Give Amina an intramuscular injection of **benzylpenicillin** (0.1 million IU for each kg of body weight up to 2 million IU) and **send** her immediately **to hospital**.

Epiglottitis

Hassan, a 3-year-old boy, has been ill since yesterday. He has a fever and is **not able to eat or drink**. He is leaning forward and has a lot of saliva coming out of his mouth. Hassan has epiglottitis. **Do not look at** Hassan's **throat**.

Treatment: Give Hassan an intramuscular injection of **chloramphenicol** (40 mg for each kg of body weight up to 1000 mg) or **benzylpenicillin** and **send** him immediately **to hospital**.

Mouth pain

POSTER 5:
(Summary poster)

How to treat mouth problems

If a patient has pain in the mouth **press on** the **teeth**:
- If **one of the teeth** is **painful** when you touch it, treat the patient for a **tooth abscess**. A tooth abscess can be caused by tooth decay. Tooth decay happens if a person does not brush his teeth twice a day and does not eat a good mixed diet. Treat a tooth abscess with **metronidazole 200 mg three times a day for 5 days** or phenoxymethylpenicillin, at the normal dose, for 5 days. **Send** the patient **to** see a **dentist**.

Look at the **gums**:
- If the gums are painful, or blood comes from the gums, the patient may have **gingivitis** or an **ulcer in his mouth**. Gingivitis and mouth ulcers are caused by, or made worse by, a bad diet and not brushing the teeth. **Advise** the patient to eat a **mixed diet** and to **brush his teeth and to wash out his mouth with clean salted water twice a day**. He should not use sea water.

Ask one of the students to show the class how to make a toothbrush. Make a toothbrush from soft wood, for example the stalk of a banana tree. Use a knife to cut away the outer parts of the stalk. Next, bite the end of the stick until you produce a soft brush. Brush the teeth every morning and night. Use charcoal, salt or baking powder.

Oral candida

One cause of pain in the mouth is more common if a patient has HIV or malnutrition or is taking antibiotics.

Ask the students what this problem is and what it looks like. Look for the following answers:

Answer   Oral candida. This is sometimes called thrush.

Answer   You will see **white areas on top of painful red areas** inside the mouth.

Next, ask your students: What is the treatment for oral candida? Look for the following answers:

Answer   If nystatin is available, give the patient 100,000 units, after food, four times a day for 7 days. The patient should rinse the mouth and then swallow the nystatin.

Answer   Rinse the mouth with gentian violet two times a day for 7 days. Tell the patient not to swallow the gentian violet.

SECTION 3: When to refer patients to hospital

Give each student a copy of Tables 1 to 4.

TABLE 1 Ear problems

Ear problem	Treatment
Green or yellow discharge from the ear no better 7 days after starting co-trimoxazole or amoxicillin	Send to ear, nose and throat clinic
Foreign body in the ear and discharge from the ear	Send to ear, nose and throat clinic
Foreign body in the ear that cannot be removed using a syringe and water	Send to ear, nose and throat clinic
Mastoiditis or cellulitis	Procaine penicillin fortified, chloramphenicol or benzyl-penicillin and send to hospital

TABLE 2 Throat problems

Throat problems	Treatment
Diphtheria	Give an injection of benzylpenicillin. Send immediately to hospital
Epiglottitis	Do not look at the throat. Give an injection of chloramphenicol or benzylpenicillin. Send immediately to hospital

TABLE 3 Mouth problems

Mouth problem	Treatment
Oral candida	Gentian violet or nystatin for 7 days. Advise about HIV and send to an HIV counselling and testing centre
Tooth abscess	Metronidazole 200 mg three times a day for 5 days or phenoxymethylpenicillin for 5 days. Send to a dentist

TABLE 4   Nose problems

Nose problem	Treatment
Blood coming from the nose. Patient feels light-headed and the pulse is faster than 110 beats in 1 minute	Press the soft part of the nose on both sides continuously. Lean forward. Give oral rehydration solution 5 ml every minute. Send to hospital immediately
If there is still blood coming from the nose 1 hour after you started to treat the patient	Send to hospital. He should see an ear, nose and throat doctor if possible
Foreign body in the nose has not come out after he has blown hard through his nose 10 times	Send to hospital. He should see an ear, nose and throat doctor if possible

Refreshment break

SECTION 4:   Practical

Blood coming from the nose

DEMONSTRATION 1:   Ask one student to play the part of a 50-year-old woman called Damu. Ask a second student to play the doctor. Damu has blood coming from her nose. Tell the student who is playing the part of the doctor to do the following things to help Damu as you read them out:

1. Gently press the soft part of the nose on both sides for 10 minutes. Bleeding usually comes from near the front of the nose.
2. Lean Damu forward to stop blood going down the back of the throat.
3. Put something between her teeth, a pen, for example, to stop her swallowing blood. This will also help the blood to clot in the nose. If there is still bleeding 1 hour after starting treatment, send the patient to hospital, to see an ear, nose and throat doctor if possible.
4. Count how many times the pulse beats in one minute. If the patient has already lost a large amount of blood, feels light-headed and her pulse beats 110 or more times in 1 minute, she is ill with shock. Give her oral rehydration solution 5 ml every minute. Send to hospital.

5. Measure the blood pressure. High blood pressure sometimes causes blood to come from the nose. If the patient's blood pressure is 120 mmHg or more, send the patient to hospital immediately.
6. If the patient does not need to go to hospital and the bleeding stops, put some vaseline inside the nose 2 hours after blood has stopped coming out. Tell the patient to put vaseline inside the nose two times a day for 5 days. This will help the nose to heal.

Foreign body in the nose

DEMONSTRATION 2: Ask one student to play the patient, a 4-year-old boy called Fadhil. Ask another student to play the part of the doctor. For the last 2 days, pus has come out of Fadhil's left nostril. Tell the student who is playing the part of the doctor to do the following things to help Fadhil as you read them out:

1. The doctor wipes the nose. She looks up the nose. There is something hard in the left nostril.
2. Next, the doctor presses firmly on the soft part of the nostril which does not have a foreign body in it.
3. Place a cloth over the end of Fadhil's nose. Ask him to close his mouth and to blow hard through his nose.
4. If the foreign body has not come out after blowing the nose 10 times, send the patient to hospital, to see an ear, nose and throat doctor if possible.

Foreign body in the ear

- If a patient has something in his ear and there is pus coming out of the ear, send him to the ear, nose and throat clinic.
- If there is no pus, use a syringe and soapy water to take the foreign body out.

DEMONSTRATION 3: You need a syringe (5 ml or larger), a cup of water, some soap, a bowl and a towel or cloth. Ask one student play a doctor and another student to play a girl called Sita. Sita has something in her ear. There is no pus coming from her ear. Tell the student who is playing the part of the doctor to do the following things to help Sita as you read them out:

1. Put a towel or a cloth on the patient's shoulder. Put a bowl underneath the ear.
2. Put some warm soapy water in a cup.
3. Fill a syringe with warm soapy water.
4. Put the end of the syringe into the top of the ear hole. Push the syringe so that water comes out very quickly.
5. Do this several times until the foreign body has come out of the ear.
6. If the foreign body will not come out of the ear, send the patient to the ear, nose and throat clinic.

Wax blocking the ear

Wax which has been pushed against the eardrum may cause poor hearing. If a patient has poor hearing and there is no pus in the ear, treat the patient for ear wax. The following demonstration shows you how to treat ear wax.

DEMONSTRATION 4:

Ask one student to play a doctor and another student to play a patient called Thomas. Thomas has been having problems hearing recently. There is no pus coming from his ear. Tell the student who is playing the part of the doctor to do the following things to help Thomas as you read them out:

1. Advise the patient not to clean the ear with a stick. Explain that trying to clean the ear with a stick may cause permanent deafness.
2. Put three drops of vegetable oil into the ear twice a day for 5 days. Vegetable oil, such as coconut oil, makes the wax soft. When the wax is soft it is easier to remove. Often the wax and dirt will come out with no other treatment.
3. If after 2 weeks the patient still has poor hearing he should come back to the health centre. Use a syringe and soapy water to clean the ear.

SECTION 5:   Answers to the quiz

Ask the students to call out the answers to each question in the quiz.

1. A patient has a fever and a yellow or green discharge from his ear. How do you treat him?
   Give him co-trimoxazole for 5 days in malaria areas. Or give amoxicillin if the patient is pregnant or there is no malaria in your area. If the discharge is no better 1 week after starting treatment, send the patient to the ear, nose and throat clinic.

2. What are the symptoms of diphtheria? How do you treat diphtheria?
   The throat is painful. There are white or grey areas which cover the tonsils but the throat is only slightly red. Give an intramuscular injection of benzylpenicillin and send immediately to hospital.

3. What are the symptoms of epiglottitis? How do you treat epiglottitis?
   The throat is painful. The patient is not able to drink. Do not examine the throat. Give an intramuscular injection of chloramphenicol or benzylpenicillin. Send the patient to hospital immediately.

Eye problems

BEFORE THE LESSON

■ There are four posters in this lesson. (See p. 4 for information on how to use the posters.) Prepared posters: 1, 2, 3, 4

■ Prepare one copy of Appendix 21 for each student.

■ You need some thin sticks, thin cardboard, pins and scissors for the practicals in section 3.

■ Draw large copies of Pictures 38, 39, 40, 41, 42, 43, 44, 46, 47, 48, 49 and 51 of 12 eye problems. Do not label the pictures. Give these pictures to students for the practical in section 4.

SECTION 1: Quiz

POSTER 1:
(Prepared poster)

Quiz

Ask the students to answer the questions on their own. Do not give the answers until the end of the lesson.

> 1. A 2-week-old baby has had pus coming out of both eyes for 2 days. What could cause this?
> 2. Name three causes of pain in the eye.
> 3. Name three causes of poor eyesight when the eye is not red.
> 4. A patient has a red eye which is painful. Her eyesight in that eye is worse than normal. How will you treat her?

SECTION 2: Information about the eyes

In developing countries, most types of blindness can be prevented or cured. For example, we can prevent blindness caused by lack of vitamin A deficiency and we can treat cataracts. Today you will learn how to identify and treat common and important eye problems.

If you know what a healthy eye looks like, you will know when the patient has an eye problem.

POSTER 2:
(Prepared poster)

The front of a normal eye

Draw Picture 35 on Poster 2.
Point to each part of the eye and explain how it works.

• **Eyelids** close to prevent the eye from becoming dry.
• The **conjunctiva** is a clear wet skin that covers the white part of the eye and the inside of the eyelids.

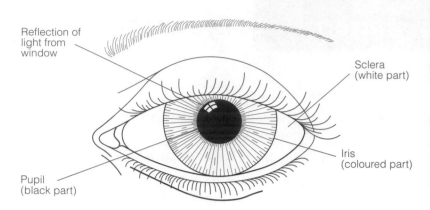

Reflection of light from window

Sclera (white part)

Iris (coloured part)

Pupil (black part)

PICTURE 35 *The front of a normal eye*

- The black **pupil** gets bigger at night to let in more light. The coloured **iris** is a circle of muscle that changes size to make the black pupil bigger.
- Behind the black pupil is a clear piece of jelly called the **lens**. The lens allows us to see both things that are near to us and things that are far away from us.
- The **cornea** is the window of the eye in front of the black pupil and coloured iris.

SECTION 3: Practical: How to examine the eye

Show students how to make a multiple pin-hole occluder. You will need thin cardboard, several small pins, several pairs of scissors. Copy picture 36 of an occluder with five pin-holes. Make the occluder 21 cm long and the pin-holes approximately 8 mm apart in a cross.

Put a pin through the card in these 5 places to make holes

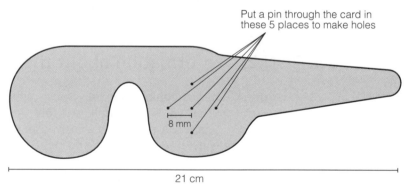

8 mm

21 cm

PICTURE 36 *Multiple pin-hole occluder*

Ask a student volunteer to stand with you at the front of the class. Examine the volunteer's eye as shown in Picture 37. Slowly show the other students how to examine the eye. Explain how to examine the eye.

1. The patient should sit facing a window.

2. Look at the eyelids.

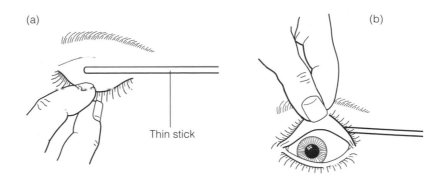

(a)

Thin stick

(b)

PICTURE 37 *How to examine the upper eyelid*

- Put a finger on the lower eyelid and gently pull it down. Look at the inside of the eyelid.
- If the patient has pain in the eye, also look under the upper eyelid. Put a thin stick on the upper eyelid. Hold the stick with your left hand to examine the right eye. With the fingers of your other hand gently pull the eyelashes down. Ask the patient to look down. Lift the eyelid so that it folds over the stick. Wipe the inside of the eyelid with a clean soft cloth or cotton wool.

3. Look at the white part of the eye.
   - Is it the normal colour?
   - Is the white part of the eye more red than usual?
   - Is the area next to the cornea most red?

4. Look at the cornea and the iris. In a healthy eye, the cornea is clear with no marks on it and you can see the iris clearly.

5. Look at the pupil. Normal pupils are black and the same size.

6. Finally, ask the patient if his eyesight, **in that eye**, is worse than usual. Put the pin-holes of the occluder directly in front of the bad eye. Cover the good eye completely. Ask the patient if he can see better or read better through the little holes. If the patient is a child, ask the patient to pick up a small object.

Ask the students to sit together in pairs and to practise examining each other's eyes. Give one stick each to two students. Observe them and make sure they know how to do this correctly.

If after examining a patient's eyes you still do not know why a patient has poor eyesight:
1. look for a fever
2. look for anaemia
3. measure the blood pressure
4. test a urine sample for sugar (to see if the patient has diabetes). You may need to send the patient to hospital for this test.

Fever, anaemia, high blood pressure or diabetes may cause poor eyesight.

SECTION 4: Diagnosis and management

Symptoms and signs

Give each student a copy of Appendix 21. Explain how to use Appendix 21:

Column 1 of Appendix 21 tells you about the three groups of eye problems:
1. red eye or eyes
2. poor eyesight when the eye is not red
3. swelling next to the eye.

You use column 1 of Appendix 21 to decide which type of eye problems your patient has.

Column 2 tells you the questions you need to ask to find out about the main symptoms and signs of the eye problem. If the answer to *any* question in column 2 is 'yes', look at the group diagnosis in column 3.

Next, look for the other symptoms and signs for that group diagnosis in column 4. When you find the symptom or sign that your patient has, you can make a full diagnosis.

The treatment for each diagnosis is described in column 5.

Tell the students that they will now use Appendix 21 to identify 19 eye problems in the following examples.

Give the pictures of eye problems to 12 students. Explain that each picture shows a different eye problem.

Next, tell the students that you will describe patients with symptoms and signs of different eye problems. The students should use Appendix 21 to decide which eye problem each patient has. If a student thinks that her picture shows that eye problem, she will stand up and tell the class why her picture shows that eye problem. Tell the students that it does not matter if they get it wrong.

Red eye

Group diagnosis 1: Painful red eye

Eye problem 1: Iritis
Amina is a 30-year-old woman. She has had pain in her left eye since yesterday. Amina does not have any other illness. Amina's eyelids are normal. The white part of the eye is more red than usual. The white part of the eye next to the cornea is very red. The cornea looks cloudy. The left pupil is smaller than the right pupil. Amina tells you she *cannot* see well with her left eye. Amina has iritis. Iritis is caused by an allergy. Amina's symptoms and signs could also be caused by a corneal ulcer.

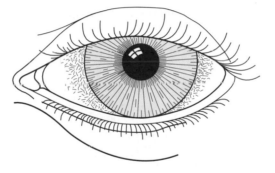

PICTURE 38 *Eye problem 1: iritis*

Ask the students: 'Does your picture show iritis? Why?'

Treatment: Put tetracycline eye ointment in the eye. Give Amina an intramuscular injection of benzylpenicillin and send her to hospital immediately. If the patient is a child less than 6 years old, give vitamin A.

Eye problem 2: Corneal ulcer

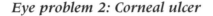

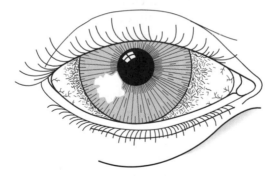

PICTURE 39 *Eye problem 2: corneal ulcer*

Maulidi is a 52-year-old man. He has had pain and a large amount of water coming out of his right eye for 3 days. Maulidi does not have any other illness. His eyelids look normal. The white part of the eye next to the cornea is very red. There is a mark on the cornea. The pupil is black. Maulidi tells you he cannot see well with his right eye. Maulidi has a corneal ulcer.

Ask the students: 'Does your picture show a corneal ulcer? Why?'

Treatment: Put tetracycline eye ointment in the right eye and give an intramuscular injection of benzylpenicillin. Next, send Maulidi to hospital immediately. Corneal ulcers may be caused by herpes virus, bacteria or fungus infections, or by lack of vitamin A. Give vitamin A if a patient is less than 6 years old.

Eye problem 3: Acute glaucoma

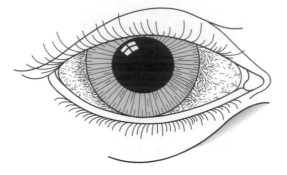

PICTURE 40 *Eye problem 3: acute glaucoma*

Mosi is a 50-year-old woman. Her right eye is red. Mosi has had severe pain in her right eye for 2 hours. She does not have any other illness. The eyelids are normal. The white part of the eye next to the cornea is very red. There is a large amount of water coming out of the eye. The cornea is not clear. The right pupil is bigger than the left pupil. The pupil is not black because the cornea is not clear. Mosi cannot see well with the right eye. Mosi has acute glaucoma. A corneal ulcer can cause the same symptoms and signs.

Ask the students: 'Does your picture show acute glaucoma? Why?'

Treatment: Put tetracycline eye ointment in the right eye. Give Mosi an intramuscular injection of benzylpenicillin and send her to the eye hospital immediately. Give vitamin A if a patient is less than 6 years old.

Eye problem 4: Corneal foreign body

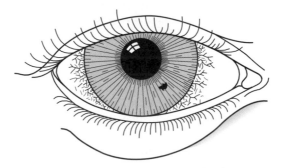

PICTURE 41 *Eye problem 4: corneal foreign body*

Hassan is a 32-year-old man. Yesterday, he felt something go into his right eye. Hassan was not able to sleep because of pain. Hassan does not have any other illness. The insides of the eyelids are normal. The white part of the eye next to the cornea is red. There is a large amount of water coming out of the eye. You can see a small black object on the cornea. The pupil is black. Hassan says that he can see well with his right eye but that it is difficult to keep the eye open. Hassan has a foreign body in his cornea or a corneal abrasion.

Ask the students: 'Does your picture show a corneal foreign body? Why?'

Treatment: Try to wash the foreign body out of the eye with clean water. Wipe the inside of the upper eyelid. Put tetracycline eye ointment in the eye. If the eye is still painful, send the patient to hospital immediately.

Some foreign bodies go fast enough to go inside the eye. If the patient was using a hammer or chisel, or cannot see well following an accident, or there is blood behind the cornea, send him to an eye hospital immediately.

Group diagnosis 2: Irritated red eye. No pain. Eyesight is normal

Eye problem 5: Viral conjunctivitis

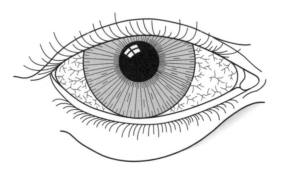

PICTURE 42 *Eye problem 5: viral conjunctivitis*

Two children, Ali aged 3 years and Saidi aged 5 years, have runny noses and irritated eyes. Ali and Saidi do not have any other illness. In both children, the inside of the eyelids are very red. The white part of the eye is more red than usual. The cornea is clear. The pupil is black. Saidi and Ali are able to pick up a pen easily. Ali and Saidi have viral conjunctivitis. With viral conjunctivitis, there is little or no pus and the eyes are red for less than 7 days. Measles is a virus that can cause conjunctivitis.

Ask the students: 'Does your picture show viral conjunctivitis? Why?'

Treatment: Tell the patients (or the mother) to wash their faces and hands three or four times a day. Each child should not use the same towel as anyone else. Tell the mother to bring the children back if their eyes are no better after 7 days.

A patient with measles has a rash on his body and a fever. If you think a child may have measles, treat him with vitamin A. Vitamin A prevents serious eye problems and death in children. Give the first dose of vitamin A at the health centre. If a child has fever and there is malaria in the area, give the first line malaria treatment.

Eye problem 6: Bacterial conjunctivitis

Conjunctivitis may also be caused by bacterial infection. A patient has bacterial conjunctivitis if there is a large amount of pus in the eye and the eye has been red for less than 7 days.

Treatment: Give tetracycline eye ointment two times a day for 5 days. Tell the patient to go to the eye hospital if he is no better after 3 days.

Eye problem 7: Trachoma or allergic conjunctivitis

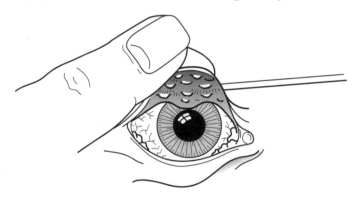

PICTURE 43 *Eye problem 7: trachoma or allergic conjunctivitis*

Asha is 11 years old. Both of her eyes are red and irritated. Ten days ago, Asha was given tetracycline eye ointment. Asha does not have any other illness. You turn Asha's top eyelids inside out. There are many small swellings on the inside of the eyelids. The white part of the eye is more red than usual. There is a small amount of pus in her eyes. The cornea is clear. The pupil is black. Asha tells you that she can see well.

Asha may have conjunctivitis caused by trachoma or an allergy to the eye ointment. If conjunctivitis is no better 7 days after starting eye ointment, it may be caused by an allergy to eye ointment. Stop the eye ointment.

If conjunctivitis is no better 3 days after stopping eye ointment, it is probably caused by trachoma. Trachoma is passed from person to person on dirty fingers and by flies.

It causes mild conjunctivitis which continues for a long time. If a patient has many trachoma infections over many years, trachoma can scar the eyelids. These scars may cause the eyelids to bend and to rub against the cornea. If the cornea is damaged it will become scarred and white. Corneal scarring causes blindness.

Ask the students 'Does your picture show trachoma or allergic conjunctivitis? Why?'

Treatment: Tell Asha to stop using the eye ointment, she may have allergic conjunctivitis. Tell her to go to the eye clinic if she is no better after 3 days. Trachoma is treated with tetracycline eye ointment for at least 6 weeks. Normally an eye nurse or doctor will start this treatment. Washing the face and eyes two times a day can prevent trachoma. Using latrines and burying rubbish will reduce the number of flies. There is no treatment for corneal scarring.

Eye problem 8: Gonococcal conjunctivitis

Pili was born less than 5 days ago. Pili has a large amount of pus coming out of both eyes. Her eyelids are swollen. Pili does not have any other illness. The inside of the eyelids are very red. The white parts of the eyes are more red than usual. The corneas are clear. The pupils are black. Pili has gonococcal conjunctivitis.

Treatment: Put tetracycline ointment in both eyes six times a day for 5 days. Give Pili the first-line treatment for gonorrhoea, or intramuscular injections of procaine penicillin fortified once a day, or intramuscular benzylpenicillin two times each day, for 5 days. Tell the mother that Pili was infected with gonococcal conjunctivitis during birth. This can happen to a baby if the mother has gonorrhoea. Tell the parents that they have gonorrhoea, which is a sexually transmitted disease. Send the mother and father to the sexually transmitted disease clinic.

Eye problem 9: Chlamydia conjunctivitis

If a baby is more than 5 days old but less than 1 month old and has pus coming out of the eyes, the baby may have chlamydia conjunctivitis. A baby is infected with chlamydia conjunctivitis during birth if the mother has chlamydia infection.

Ask the students 'Does your picture show conjunctivitis which could be caused by gonorrhoea or chlamydia? Why?' The correct picture is the picture of viral conjunctivitis but there must also be pus in the eyes for gonococcal or chlamydia conjunctivitis.

Treatment: Put tetracycline ointment in the eyes once a day for 3 weeks. Also give the baby erythromycin (liquid or crushed tablets) 10 mg for each kg of body weight, four times a day for 3 weeks. Tell the parents that they may have chlamydia, and send them to the sexually transmitted disease clinic.

Group diagnosis 3: Red eye. No irritation. No pain. Eyesight is normal

Eye problem 10: Sub-conjunctival haemorrhage

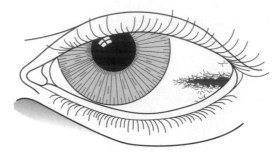

PICTURE 44 *Eye problem 10: sub-conjunctival haemorrhage*

Tracey has just given birth. There is a small collection of blood in the white part of Tracey's left eye. Her eye is not painful. Tracey does not have any other illness. The insides of the eyelids are normal. The cornea is clear. The pupil is black. Tracey is able to see well with her left eye. Her blood pressure is normal. Tracey has a sub-conjunctival haemorrhage. Small accidents, coughing, giving birth, or high blood pressure may cause a small amount of blood to collect under the conjunctiva in front of the white part of the eye.

Ask the students 'Does your picture show a sub-conjunctival haemorrhage. Why?'

Treatment: Tell the patient that the sub-conjunctival haemorrhage will go away after 2 or 3 weeks. Do not give any medicine.

Refreshment break

Poor eyesight, eye not red

Group diagnosis 4: Needs glasses or hand lens

Eye problem 11: Needs glasses or hand lens
Salim, a 50-year-old teacher, has found it difficult to read his books for the last 2 years. Salim does not have any other illness. The eyelids and the white part of the eye are normal. The cornea is clear. The pupil is black. You ask Salim to look at a book through multiple pin-holes in daylight. Salim tells you that he can read through the pin-holes. The lenses in Salim's eyes are old. Salim needs glasses or a hand lens to help him to read.

Treatment: Refer Salim to the eye clinic where he may be able to get glasses.

**Group diagnosis 5:
Possibly cross-eyed**

Eye problem 12: Cross-eyed

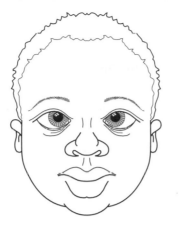

PICTURE 45 *Eye problem 12: cross-eyes*

Abduli is a 3-year-old boy. His eyes always look in different directions. Abduli does not have any other illness. The eyelids and the white parts of the eyes are normal. The corneas are clear. The pupils are black. Abduli is able to pick up a pen if you cover the left or the right eye.

Do the light reflection test. Abduli looks towards the window. You look at the reflections of the window on Abduli's corneas. You compare the positions of the reflections on Abduli's corneas with the position of the pupils. You decide that Abduli is cross-eyed, because the reflections on his corneas are in different places.

POSTER 3:
(Prepared poster)

Draw Picture 45 on Poster 3. Show students the features of cross-eyes.

Treatment: Send Abduli to the eye clinic.

**Group diagnosis 6:
Poor eyesight at night**

Eye problem 13: Lack of vitamin A

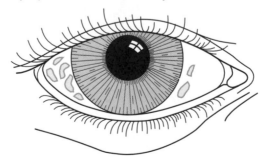

PICTURE 46 *Eye problem 13: Bitot's spots*

Siti is a 4-year-old girl. She cannot see well at night and often has accidents when it is dark. Siti does not have any other illness.

199

The eyelids and the white parts of the eyes are normal. The corneas are clear. There are dry areas on the corneas. The pupils are black. You give Siti your pen. Siti is able to pick up your pen. Siti's brother Usiku is 5 years old. He has little bubbles on either side of the cornea. These are called Bitot's spots. Siti and Usiku both have night blindness. This is caused by a lack of vitamin A.

Ask the students: 'Does your picture show lack of vitamin A? Why?' Ask the student who has a picture of a normal eye to stand up also.

Tell the students that it takes some time for lack of vitamin A to affect the eyes. If the patient has early vitamin A deficiency, the eye will look normal except for dry areas on the cornea. It is important to look carefully at the cornea if you think a patient may lack vitamin A.

Treatment: Give Siti and Usiku three doses of vitamin A:
- Give the first dose today.
- Give the second dose tomorrow.
- Give the third dose on day 14.

For children aged less than 1 year, give three doses of 100,000 IU. For children aged more than one year, give three doses of 200,000 IU.

Tell the mother about foods that contain vitamin A. Explain that her children need to eat these foods. Orange fruits and vegetables, and dark green leafy vegetables provide vitamin A. There is also some vitamin A in breastmilk.

Group diagnosis 7: Poor eyesight day and night

Eye problem 14: Cataract

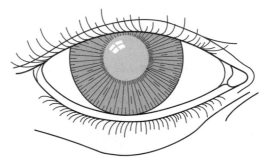

PICTURE 47 *Eye problem 14: cataract*

Rashid, a 70-year-old man, has had poor eyesight for many years. His eyesight is slowly getting worse. Rashid does not have any other illness. The insides of the eyelids are normal and the white parts of the eyes are normal. The corneas are clear. The pupils are cloudy white. You hold up your fingers 3 metres in front of Rashid and ask him to tell you how many fingers he can see. He cannot see your fingers. Rashid has cataracts. As the lenses in the eyes get old or damaged, they become cloudy white. A cloudy white lens is called a cataract.

Ask the students: 'Does your picture show a cataract? Why?'

Treatment: A short operation can sometimes cure cataracts. Tell Rashid that there is an operation which may allow him to see again. The operation is sometimes free and is not painful. Tell Rashid to go to the eye clinic.

Eye problem 15: Corneal scar from trachoma or onchocerciasis

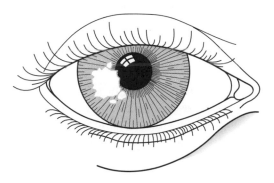

PICTURE 48 *Eye problem 15: corneal scar*

Justine is a 30-year-old woman. Her eyesight is slowly getting worse. Justine does not have any other illness. The eyelids are scarred but the white parts of the eyes are normal. Part of the cornea is white. The pupil is not black because the cornea is not clear. Justine is able to count your fingers from 3 metres but she cannot see well enough to read. Justine has a corneal scar, caused by repeated infections with trachoma.

Onchocerciasis can also damage the cornea or the iris or the back of the eye. Onchocerciasis is only seen in a few countries. The flies which give people onchocerciasis live in fast-flowing rivers.

Ask the students: 'Does your picture show a corneal scar? Why?'

Treatment: If the eye is painful, put tetracycline eye ointment in the eye and send Justine to hospital immediately. If Justine lives in an onchocerciasis area treat her and all the people in her village with ivermectin. Give ivermectin 6 mg one time every year.

Eye problem 16: Chronic glaucoma
A patient with chronic glaucoma finds it more and more difficult to see things on each side of him. After a time, the patient can only see things which are directly in front of him. Chronic

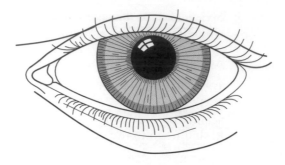

PICTURE 49 *Eye problem 16: normal eye*

glaucoma does not cause pain. The eyes look normal. Often someone else in the family is blind because of chronic glaucoma.

Ask the students: 'Could your picture show chronic glaucoma? Why?'

Treatment: Chronic glaucoma is treated with a simple operation or with eye drops every day for the rest of the patient's life. Everyone in the patient's family should go to the eye clinic when they reach the age of 40.

Swellings next to the eye

Eye problem 17: Orbital cellulitis
Ravi, a 4-year-old child, has a swollen and painful left eye. Ravi has a fever. The top and bottom eyelids of the left eye are swollen. The white part of the eye is red and swollen. The cornea is clear. The pupil is black. Ravi is able to see with his left eye but can only look forwards. Ravi has orbital cellulitis.

Treatment: Put tetracycline ointment in his eye. You give Ravi an intramuscular injection of benzylpenicillin and send him to hospital immediately.

Eye problem 18: Acute dacrocystitis

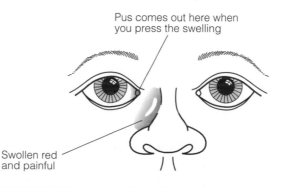

Pus comes out here when you press the swelling

Swollen red and painful

PICTURE 50 *Eye problem 18: acute dacrocystitis*

Mwanaasha, a 40-year-old woman, has pain underneath her right eye. Pus has been coming out of her eye for 2 days. Mwanaasha does not have any other illness. The eyelids are normal. The white part of the eye is red. The cornea is clear. The pupil is black. Mwanaasha can see as normal with her left eye. There is a red swelling next to the nose. When you touch the swelling, pus comes out of the eye and Mwanaasha tells you that it makes the pain worse. Mwanaasha has acute dacrocystitis.

POSTER 4:
(Prepared poster)

Draw Picture 50 on Poster 4. Show students the symptoms of acute dacrocystitis.

Treatment: Give phenoxymethylpenicillin 500 mg three times a day for 5 days. Give a lower dose if the patient weighs less than 40 kg (see dosages in Appendix 21). Also tell the patient to press the swelling, from the bottom to the top, three times a day. Tell the patient to go to the eye hospital if the eye is not better after 5 days.

Eye problem 19: Stye or infected meibomian cyst

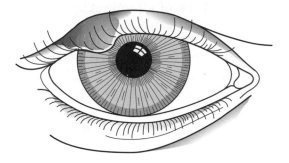

PICTURE 51 *Eye problem 19: stye or infected meibomian cyst*

Eight-year-old Suleiman has had a swelling above his right eye for 4 days. Suleiman does not have any other illness. There is a red swelling in his right eyelid near to the eyelashes. The swelling is painful when you touch it. The white part of the eye is normal. The cornea is clear. The pupil is black. Suleiman is able to see as normal with his right eye. Suleiman has a stye or an infected meibomian cyst.

Ask the students: 'Could your picture show a stye or infected meibomian cyst? Why?'

Treatment: Give Suleiman's mother tetracycline eye ointment to put in his right eye two times a day for 5 days. Tell her to take Suleiman to the eye clinic if he is not better after a week.

SECTION 5: When to refer patients to hospital

Ask the students to use Appendix 21 to tell you which patients to send to an eye hospital or clinic.

SECTION 6:   Answers to the quiz

Ask the students to call out the answers to each question in the quiz.

1. A 2-week-old baby has had pus coming out of both eyes for 2 days. What could cause this?
   Chlamydia conjunctivitis

2. Name three causes of pain in the eye.
   Corneal ulcer
   Iritis
   Acute glaucoma
   Foreign body in the cornea or corneal abrasion
   Orbital cellulitis
   Acute dacrocystitis
   Stye or infected meibomian cyst

3. Name three causes of poor eyesight when the eye is not red.
   Needs glasses
   Lack of vitamin A
   Cataract
   Chronic glaucoma
   Corneal scar from trachoma or onchocerciasis

4. A patient has a red eye which is painful. Her eyesight in that eye is worse than normal. How will you treat her?
   Put tetracycline eye ointment in the eye.
   Give benzylpenicillin intramuscularly.
   Send to eye hospital immediately.

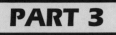

PART 3 **Appendices**

APPENDIX 1　How to treat children aged 5 years or less, who have a cough or difficult breathing

1. Questions

Ask the mother:
1. When did the symptoms **start?**
2. Has he had a **fever?**
3. Does he have a **cough or difficult breathing?**
4. Is he **feeding** and **drinking** well!?
5. Does he have **diarrhoea?**
6. What **medicines** has he had in the last 2 weeks?

2. Check for general danger signs

General danger signs:
1. If the patient is unconscious or moves less usual when awake.
2. If the patient has had a convulsion.
3. If the patient has vomited four times or more this morning.
4. If the child is not able to drink or breastfeed.

3. Diagnose and treat general danger signs

Treat general danger signs:
1. If he has vomited, clear his mouth, lay him on his side. Treat fever with tepid sponging.
2. If he is still having a convulsion give him diazepam rectally.
3. Treat to prevent low blood sugar.
4. Give him an intramuscular injection of quinine or chloroquine in malaria areas.
5. Give him an intramuscular injection of chloramphenicol, benzylpenicillin or procaine penicillin fortified.
6. **Send him to hospital** immediately.

4. Examination

There is chest indrawing

Count how many times he breathes in one minute

Look for fever and anaemia

Listen for a noise when the child breathes **in**

Listen for a noise when the child breathes **out**

5. Check symptoms then diagnose and treat

A child less than 2 months old breathes 60 times or more in one minute

A child aged 2 months or more but less than 12 months breathes 50 times or more in one minute

A child aged 12 months up to 5 years breathes 40 times or more in one minute

The child does not have fast breathing. When the child is calm there is no noise when the child breathes in

There is a hard noise when the child is calm and breathes in. He has stridor. Give him chloramphenicol. **Send him to hospital immediately**

There is a soft whistling noise when he breathes out, or it is difficult to breathe out. **He has a wheeze**

A severe illness which may be pneumonia or asthma
Give an injection of benzylpenicillin.
If has fever give an injection of quinine or chloroquine in malaria areas. If has a wheeze give a rapid acting bronchodilator. **Send to hospital**

Pneumonia which is not yet severe
Give co-trimoxazole if child has had a fever. Use amoxicillin if in an area where there is no malaria or there is no fever. Teach mother about home treatment for chest illnesses.
See again after 2 days. If no better give benzylpenicillin and **send to hospital**

No pneumonia
1. Treat wheeze if has wheeze.
2. Upper respiratory infection. If has no ear or throat problem do not give an antibiotic. Teach mother about home treatment for chest illnesses.
3. Fever. Treat for malaria in malaria areas.

Home treatment for chest illnesses:
1. Give plenty of fluids.
2. Continue feeding at least five times a day.
3. Tell mother when to return:
   (a) If the child is not able to drink or breastfeed.
   (b) If the breathing becomes difficult or fast.
   (c) If the patient becomes more ill.
   (d) If the patient develops a fever.

How to treat wheeze:
1. If has a sign of respiratory distress give a rapid acting bronchodilator, an injection of benzylpenicillin and **send to hospital.**
2. If has no sign of respiratory distress but has fast breathing treat for pneumonia which is not yet severe.
3. If has no signs of respiratory distress and does not have fast breathing give him a bronchodilator to use at home and teach mother about home treatment for chest illnesses.

APPENDIX 2 How to treat patients aged 6 years or more, who have a cough or difficult breathing

1. Questions

1. When did the symptoms **start?**
2. Have you had a **fever?**
3. Do you have a **cough?**
4. Are you eating and **drinking well?**
5. Do you have **diarrhoea?**
6. What **medicines** have you used in the last 2 weeks?
7. Cough. Point to the place where it causes pain.
8. If 13 years or more: What colour is your sputum?

2. Check for general danger signs

General danger signs:
1. If the patient is unconscious or moves less than usual when awake.
2. If the patient has had a convulsion.
3. If the patient has vomited four times or more this morning.
4. If the patient is not able to drink.

3. Diagnose and treat general danger signs

Treat general danger signs:
1. If she has vomited, clear her mouth, lay her on her side. Treat fever with tepid sponging.
2. If she is still having a convulsion give her diazepam rectally.
3. Treat to prevent low blood sugar.
4. Give her an intramuscular injection of quinine or chloroquine in malaria areas.
5. Give her an intramuscular injection of chloramphenicol, benzylpenicillin or procaine penicillin fortified.
6. **Send her to hospital** immediately.

Home treatment for chest illnesses:
1. Give plenty of fluids.
2. Eat at least four times a day.
3. Tell when to return:
   (a) If not able to drink.
   (b) If the breathing becomes difficult or fast.
   (c) If the patient becomes more ill.
   (d) If the patient develops a fever.

4. Examination

There is chest indrawing.

There is pain in the side of the chest when she coughs and there is a crackle when she breathes in when you listen with a stethoscope

Count how many times she breathes in one minute

Look for fever and anaemia

Listen for a noise when the patient breathes **in**

Listen for a noise when the patient breathes **out**

5. Check symptoms then diagnose and treat

A child aged 6 years up to 12 years old, breathes 30 times or more in one minute

A patient aged 13 years or more breathes 25 times or more in one minute.

The patient does not have fast breathing. When the patient breathes in there is no noise. There are no crackles

There is a hard noise when the patient is calm and breathes in. She has stridor. Give her chloramphenicol. **Send her to hospital immediately**

There is a soft whistling noise when she breathes out, or it is difficult to breathe out. She has a wheeze

A severe illness which may be pneumonia or asthma
Give an injection of benzylpenicillin.
If has fever give an injection of quinine or chloroquine in malaria areas. If has wheeze give a rapid acting bronchodilator.
Send to hospital

Pneumonia which is not yet severe
Give amoxicillin or co-trimoxazole.
Teach about home treatment for chest illnesses.
See again after 2 days:
1. If better but has fever give first line antimalarial in malaria areas (not if using co-trimoxazole).
2. If no better give benzylpenicillin and **send to hospital**

No pneumonia
1. Treat wheeze if it has wheeze.
2. Bronchitis. If aged 13 or more and has had green sputum for 8 days.
3. Upper respiratory infection. If has no ear or throat problem do not give an antibiotic. Teach the mother about home treatment for chest illnesses.
4. Fever. Treat for malaria in malaria area.

How to treat bronchitis:
Treat with amoxicillin 250 mg three times a day for 5 days (or co-trimoxazole in malaria areas). If has red sputum or is no better after treatment send to **TB** clinic or examine sputum for acid fast bacilli.

How to treat wheeze:
1. If has a sign of respiratory distress give a rapid acting bronchodilator, an injection of benzylpenicillin and **send to hospital.**
2. If has no sign of respiratory distress but has fast breathing treat for pneumonia which is not yet severe.
3. If has no signs of respiratory distress and does not have fast breathing give her a bronchodilator to use at home and teach the mother about home management for chest illnesses.

APPENDIX 3   How to give injections

Do not give injections if there is a safer way of giving medicine. If you give medicines by injection, you will use two types of injection:

- **Intramuscular injections** – for example, these are used to give many antibiotics, malaria treatments, ergometrine to prevent or treat postpartum haemorrhage, epinephrine to treat anaphylaxis.
- **Subcutaneous injections** – for example, these are used to give epinephrine to treat respiratory distress.

Before the injection

1. Clean your hands with soap or ash, and water.
2. Use a new or sterile needle and syringe.
3. Do not touch the metal end of the needle.
4. Learn how to draw up each medicine.
5. Put the needle and syringe together and draw up the medicine.
6. Ask the patient to sit or lie down.
7. Clean the skin at the injection site with alcohol or soap and water.

How to give intramuscular injections

Give intramuscular injections into the front outer part of the upper leg as shown in Picture 52. Do not inject into the buttocks.

If you are injecting more than 3 ml, inject half of the medicine into each leg.

1. Put the needle into the muscle.
2. Pull the plunger gently. If blood enters the syringe take the needle out and put it in at another clean area.
3. If no blood enters the syringe, inject the medicine slowly.
4. Remove the needle and clean the skin.

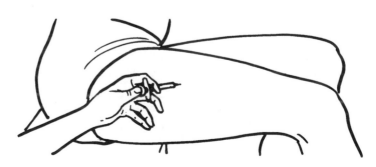

PICTURE 52   *How to give an intramuscular injection*

How to give subcutaneous injections

Give subcutaneous injections into the back of the upper arm as shown in Picture 53.

1. Hold the fatty part of the back of the upper arm with one hand.
2. Point the needle upwards so that it goes into the fat, *not* the muscle.

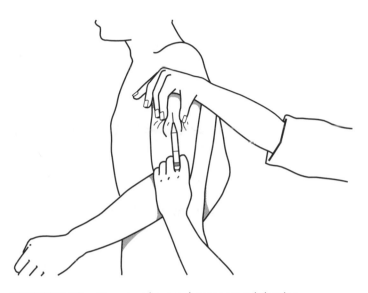

PICTURE 53 *How to give a subcutaneous injection*

After the injection

Sterilise the needle and syringe immediately after use:

1. Push bleach or soapy water through the needle and syringe three times.
2. Take everything apart.
3. Steam or boil the syringe and needle for 20 minutes. (*Note*: at altitudes over 2000 m boil for 40 minutes.)
4. Leave the syringe and needle covered until you use them again.

APPENDIX 4 How to give diazepam rectally

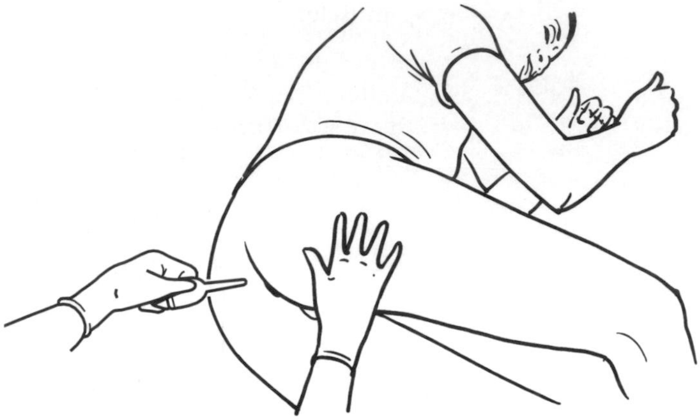

PICTURE 54 *How to give diazepam rectally*

1. Lay the patient on his left side
2. Ask the patient to bend his knees up so that they touch his abdomen.
3. Wet the end of the diazepam rectal tube with water.
4. Put the end of the rectal tube into the anus (Picture 54).
5. Push the tube gently into the rectum.
6. Squeeze the diazepam into the rectum.

APPENDIX 5   How to make a measuring bottle for liquid medicines

It is important to give the correct amount of medicine.
- If we give our patients too little medicine they will not get better.
- If we give our patients too much medicine we will not have enough medicine for other patients.

Making a measuring bottle

If you do not have a way of measuring liquid medicine, you can make a measuring bottle. You will need:
- a syringe
- a clear narrow bottle that is big enough to contain the largest amount of liquid medicine that you will measure
- tape or a pen with permanent ink to mark the side of the bottle
- liquid medicine.

Measuring the medicine

1. Decide which medicine you will measure with this bottle.
2. Decide what amounts of liquid you will need to measure for this medicine. For example, for co-trimoxazole, you will need to measure 25 ml for children aged 6 months or less, and 50 ml for children aged 7 months up to 5 years.
3. Use the syringe to put 25 ml of liquid into the bottle.
4. Make a mark at the top of the liquid.
5. Write 25 ml next to the mark.
6. Use the syringe to put a further 25 ml of liquid into the bottle.
7. Make a mark at the top of the liquid.
8. Write 50 ml next to this mark.

APPENDIX 6 How to treat malnutrition and anaemia

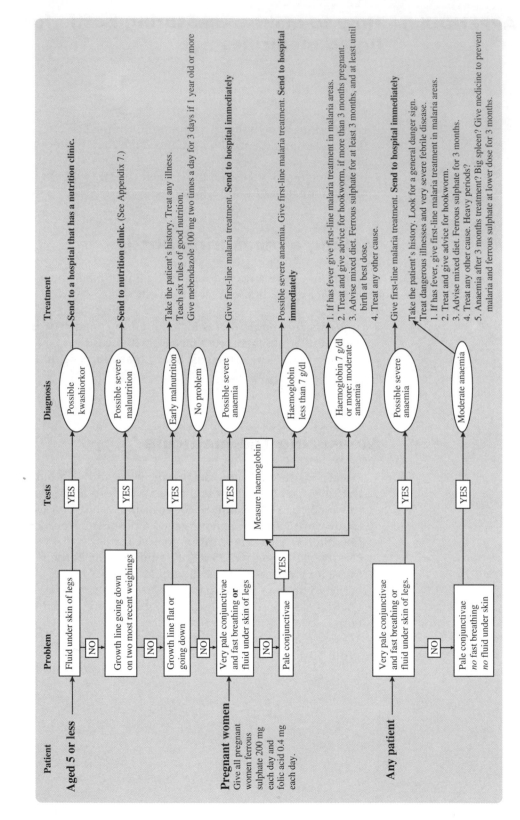

APPENDIX 7 How to set up a nutrition clinic

A nutrition clinic needs:

- a microscope and staff with the skills to examine blood and faeces to look for parasites
- a method of measuring haemoglobin and blood sugar
- trained staff to teach mothers how to grow and prepare foods that follow the six rules of good nutrition
- trained staff to decide what treatment to give each child and to review each child every week

Examination and diagnosis of a child who may have severe malnutrition

1. Look at the child's record card to see what problems, tests and treatment the child has had.
2. Test the blood for malaria and anaemia.
3. Examine the faeces with a microscope to look for eggs of worms and other parasites.
4. Measure the child's blood sugar. If the blood sugar is 2 mmol/l or less, give the patient 50 ml of sugar water or milk immediately.
5. Make sure that the child is not cold.
6. Weigh the child without her clothes. Weigh her again twice a week. Use the same scales each time. Weigh the child at the same time of day each time. Write the weights on the child's record card.

Treatment

1. If the child has malaria parasites in the blood, treat for malaria.
2. If the child has anaemia:
   - If the haemoglobin is less than 5 g/dl, give the child a blood transfusion slowly (*in hospital*). Give 20 ml of blood for each kg of body weight. Also give one dose of furosemide 20 mg by mouth.
   - If the child has fast breathing or swelling of the legs give a blood transfusion slowly (*in hospital*).
   - Treat all patients with a haemoglobin below 10 g/dl with ferrous sulphate (or a combination of ferrous sulphate with folic acid) at the full dose for 3 months.

3. If the child has worms, treat with mebendazole. If the child is less than 1 year old, give mebendazole 50 mg two times a day for 3 days.
4. Treat any other infections.
5. Give all patients vitamin A.
6. Give multivitamins every day, if multivitamins are available.
7. Feed the child (see below).

Feeding a child with severe malnutrition

1. Make the child feel comfortable when you are feeding him. Give the child time. Use a cup and a small spoon. Try using brightly-coloured cups.
2. Ask the mother to breastfeed the child if he is 2 years old or less. Breastfeed a child with malnutrition every 2 hours. If the child is not well enough to feed from the breast, the mother can express milk into a cup by pressing the nipple between two fingers and squeezing the breast for several minutes. She should do this for both breasts every 2 hours. Feed the milk to the baby using a small spoon.
3. If the child will not feed using a cup and a spoon, put in a nasogastric tube. Use a syringe to feed the child.
4. If the mother is ill and not producing enough breastmilk, also give the child nutrition milk (see recipe below) after each breastfeed. Use a cup and a spoon
   - Do not give children who have fluid underneath their skin or a nasogastric tube too much nutrition milk, because this may cause heart failure.
   - Give children who have fluid underneath the skin or a nasogastric tube 100 ml of nutrition milk for each kg body weight in a day.
   - Make enough nutrition milk for one day. For example a child who weighs 8 kg needs 100 ml for each kg of body weight. This is a total of 800 ml in one day. Feed the child every 2 hours during the day. Give eight feeds of 100 ml each day.
   - If the child does not have fluid under the skin or a nasogastric tube, give him between 150 ml and 200 ml nutrition milk for each kg of body weight in a day.
5. Give nutrition porridge to the child as soon as the child is able to eat. Give nutrition porridge two times a day at first if the child has not been eating.
6. Give nutrition porridge four times a day as soon as the child is able to play. Give fruit and vegetables between feeds. Stop giving nutrition milk. Continue to breastfeed.
7. Next, give the child solid foods to chew. Let the child feed himself with his hands or a spoon.

Recipes

Nutrition milk

To make 1000 ml you need:

- 750 ml cows' milk or goats' milk
- 1 egg
- 6 teaspoonfuls (6 × 5 ml) of sugar
- 6 teaspoonfuls (6 × 5 ml) of cooking oil

1. Put these foods into a cooking pot and mix.
2. Heat until the food boils.
3. Stir occasionally.
4. Remove the pot from the heat and cover.
5. Let the milk cool before giving to the child.

Nutrition porridge

To make enough for one meal you need:

- 2 large spoons of ground maize, sorghum, cassava or rice
- 1 handful of peanuts, small fish or 1 egg
- 2 teaspoonfuls of sugar
- 1 teaspoonful (5 ml) of cooking oil
- 1½ cups of water

1. For children less than 1 year old, grind the peanuts or small fish.
2. Put the foods into a cooking pot and mix.
3. Heat until the food boils.
4. Stir occasionally.
5. Remove the pot from the heat and cover.
6. Let it cool a little before giving to the child.

Watch for changes

If the child is doing well:

- Her weight will start to increase.
- If the child had fluid underneath the skin, her weight may decrease before increasing. This is because the fluid underneath the skin is disappearing as the child gets better.
- The child will start to eat well, play and smile when she is better.

If the child is not doing well:

- Her weight will not increase or it may decrease.
- If the child continues to have diarrhoea, look again for an infection.
- Examine the faeces for parasites.
- Examine the urine.
- Look for TB or HIV.
- Sometimes milk will make the diarrhoea worse. Do not stop the milk.

Teach the mother

1. Start to teach the mother immediately.
   - Explain to the mother why her child is in hospital.
   - Tell the mother that you will help her to make sure her child grows.
   - Tell her that a mixed diet is the most important part of the child's treatment.
   - Tell her that you will also give her child treatment for problems which are stopping him from growing.
2. Ask respected local women to teach groups of mothers how to grow and cook nutritious foods for a mixed diet. They can show the mothers how to improve the meals they cook already.
3. Show mothers how they can follow the six rules of good nutrition.
4. Send the mother and child home:
   - when the mother knows how to feed her child
   - if the child smiles
   - when the child can eat four meals of nutrition porridge each day and can eat other solid foods.
5. Ask the mother to bring him back to the nutrition clinic after 1 month.

APPENDIX 8   Sickle cell disease

People with sickle cell disease are born with the disease, but they do not become ill before 6 months of age. Their bodies make red blood cells that do not work correctly. Without preventative treatment, children with sickle cell disease usually die before they are 4 years old. If you think that a patient may have sickle cell disease, send him to hospital for a test.

Problems and signs of sickle cell disease

Anaemia

The red blood cells of a person with sickle cell disease die more quickly than normal. Malaria and other infections can cause sickle cell disease red blood cells to die very quickly, causing anaemia. Look for and treat malaria and anaemia.

Pain and swelling of joints and bones

Sickle cell disease often causes fingers or toes to swell. Pain in the chest or abdomen is also common. This because damaged red blood cells block blood vessels and cause part of the joint, bone or other part of the body to die. The swelling is very painful. If a bone is hot or red, treat for osteomyelitis. If a joint is hot or tender treat for septic arthritis.

Frequent infections

Patients with sickle cell disease are more likely to get pneumococcal pneumonia and sinusitis.

Tall forehead

Patients with sickle cell disease make red blood cells in the front of the skull. Children with sickle cell disease who are older than 4 years have a tall forehead.

Slow growth

Children with sickle cell disease grow more slowly than other children. They are often slow to learn how to sit up and to talk.

Advice for parents of children with sickle cell disease

1. The child was born with sickle cell disease. He got the disease from both his father and his mother.
2. Any future children the couple has will have a one-in-four chance of being born with the disease.
3. This disease will not go away.
4. The child should eat a mixed diet.
5. It is very important that the child drinks plenty of fluids if he gets diarrhoea.

6. The blood is weak, so the child may be out of breath.
7. The blood may become solid inside parts of the body, causing pain in the bones, the chest or the stomach.
8. Although the disease cannot be cured, medicines will make the child stronger.
9. It is important for the child to take one 5 mg tablet of folic acid each day to make the blood stronger.
10. The child must take treatment to prevent malaria.
11. It is important to come to the health centre as soon as possible if the child is ill.
12. Get more tablets before his folic acid or malaria tablets are finished.

Preventative treatment

1. Give folic acid 5 mg every day and eat a mixed diet.
2. If possible, give the child medicine to prevent malaria. The doctor at the hospital should tell you what the first-line malaria treatment is in your country.
3. The child should sleep under a mosquito net that has been treated with an insecticide (permethrin every 6 months or deltamethrin every 12 months).
4. Tell the mother that the child must be treated very quickly if he gets malaria or other infections.
5. Do not give the child treatment with ferrous sulphate.
6. Give the child all of the normal immunisations.

Treatment when a child with sickle cell disease is ill

1. It is very important to prevent dehydration. Give the child 1 teaspoonful of oral rehydration solution every minute until he passes pale urine.
2. Give the child something to reduce pain, for example paracetamol.
3. Treat any infections immediately. If the child has a fever, treat or test for malaria immediately.
4. If the child becomes ill with severe pain, treat with:
   - oral rehydration solution
   - first-line malaria treatment
   - paracetamol
   - two times the normal dose of co-trimoxazole
   - send the child to hospital
5. The child may become severely anaemic. He will have very white conjunctivae and may breathe faster than normal. He child may have swollen legs. Give the child:
   - first-line malaria treatment
   - folic acid
   - benzylpenicillin
   - send the child to hospital. The child may need a blood transfusion.

APPENDIX 9   How to make treatments for fungus infections

These two medicines are for putting on to the skin to treat yeast or fungus infections. Do not drink these medicines. The recipes and the picture are reproduced with kind permission from the book *Natural Medicine in the Tropics*, by Dr Hans Martin-Hirt and Bindanda M'Pia.

Recipe 1

1. Press the sap (juice) out of the fresh leaves of the *Cassia alata*, the ringworm bush, using a wooden stick in a wooden pounding bowl.
2. Rub the sap on the affected area two or three times each day. Alternatively, mix the sap with the same amount of palm oil. This medicine will only keep for one day.

Recipe 2

1. Collect the white latex or sap from the skin of unripe papaya (pawpaw) fruit. Leave the fruit on the tree when you collect the sap.
2. Mix the sap as follows:
   - 10 drops of papaya latex (sap)
   - 1 handful of young fresh *Cassia alata* leaves pounded
   - 1 large spoonful of vegetable oil. Palm oil or ricinus (castor) oil are suitable.
3. Rub this mixture onto the infected area three times a day. This preparation will only keep for one day.

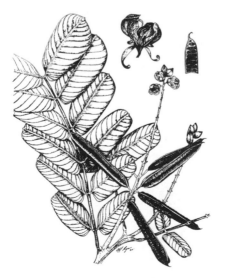

PICTURE 55   *Cassia alata*

APPENDIX 10   How to treat diarrhoea

1. Questions

1. How many times have you passed faeces this morning?
2. Do you have a fever?
3. Is there any blood in your faeces?
4. How long have you had diarrhoea?

2. Check for general danger signs

General danger signs:
1. If the patient is unconscious or moves less than usual when awake.
2. If the patient has had a convulsion.
3. If the patient has vomited four times or more this morning.
4. If the patient is not able to drink or breastfeed.

3. Diagnosis and treatment

Treat general danger signs:
1. If he has vomited, clear his mouth, lay him on his side. Treat fever with tepid sponging.
2. If he is still having a convulsion give him diazepam rectally.
3. Give oral rehydration solution 5 ml each minute.
4. Give him an intramuscular injection of quinine or chloroquine in malaria areas.
5. Give him an intramuscular injection of chloramphenicol, benzylpenicillin or procaine penicillin fortified.
6. **Send him to hospital immediately.**

Dysentery: Often only home treatment. If a child had dysentery or has malnutrition give co-trimoxazole for 5 days. If an adult is very ill, or not getting better after 5 days, give co-trimoxazole

Peritonitis: **Send to a hospital where operations are done**

4. Examination

Examine the abdomen if:
1. There is blood in the diarrhoea *or*
2. There is pain in the abdomen.

5. Findings

There is blood in the diarrhoea but the patient does not have an abdominal problem.

There is guarding or rebound tenderness.

The skin takes more than 2 seconds to become flat again. Mouth is dry

The skin goes back slowly. The skin takes less than 2 seconds to become flat again. Mouth is dry

The skin goes back quickly. Mouth is not dry

Pinch a fold of skin

6. Immediate treatment

Severe dehydration: Put in a nasogastric tube. Give **20 ml** oral rehydration solution **for each kg** body weight every hour, for **6 hours.**

Some dehydration: Give **20 ml** oral rehydration solution **for each kg** body weight every hour, for **4 hours.**

Persistent diarrhoea: Send patients who have had diarrhoea for more than 2 weeks **to hospital**
Home treatment:
1. Give as much fluid as the patient will take between feeds. Aim to make urine clear.
2. Continue feeding at least five times a day.
3. Tell mother when to return:
   (a) If the patient is not able to drink or breastfeed.
   (b) If the patient beomes more ill.
   (c) If the patient develops a fever.
   (d) If there is blood in the patient's faeces.

7. Treatment after 4–6 hours

The patient has passed very watery faeces six times or more this morning. **Send him to a cholera treatment centre.** Continue to give oral rehydration solution 5 ml each minute

Pinch a fold of skin again

If the skin takes more than 2 seconds to become flat again **send to hospital.** Continue to give oral rehydration solution 5 ml each minute.

If the skin takes less than 2 seconds to become flat again. Give **20 ml** oral rehydration solution for each kg body weight every hour, for **4 hours.**

If the skin goes back quickly. Give **home treatment** if he is able to drink. Give oral rehydration solution. Show how to make up the solution.

Fever: Treat cause of fever.

Look for fever and anaemia

220

APPENDIX 11   How to put in a nasogastric tube

1. Use a clean rubber or plastic nasogastric tube:
   - For a child use a tube 2.0 mm to 2.7 mm in diameter.
   - For an adult use a tube 4.0 mm to 6.9 mm in diameter.

2. Sit the patient down. Raise the head slightly.

3. Measure the length of tube that the patient will swallow. Place one end of the tube just above the middle of the abdomen.

4. Next, take the rest of the tube over the back of the ear and forward to the end of the nose. Mark the tube with a piece of tape where it touches the end of the nose.

5. Wet the tube with water. Do not use oil.

6. Put the end of the tube into the larger nostril. Aim towards the back of the head. Push the tube slowly until the end is in the back of the throat.

7. Ask the patient to drink a little water if the patient is awake. Each time the patient swallows, push the tube another 3 cm.

8. If the patient coughs repeatedly, pull the tube back slowly until the coughing stops. Wait a minute. Next, slowly try to push the tube again.

9. Stop when the tape marker reaches the nose.

10. Put a stethoscope (or your ear) on the upper abdomen. Use a syringe to push air quickly into the tube. Listen.
    - If the end of the tube is in the stomach you will hear air entering the stomach.
    - If you cannot hear air bubbling into the stomach do not put any fluid into the tube.
    - If you do not hear air entering the stomach check that the tube is not all at the back of the throat.
    - If the tube is not all in the throat, and the patient is not coughing, push the tube 5 cm further. Next push air into the tube again.

11. When you hear air entering the stomach fasten the tube to the face with tape.

12. Use a syringe to give oral rehydration solution, milk or sugar water.
    - Give 20 ml of fluid for each kg body weight every hour slowly throughout the hour to treat dehydration.
    - Give 30–50 ml of milk or sugar water quickly to patients with a general danger sign.

APPENDIX 12   Other treatments for diarrhoea

These are two treatments for diarrhoea which you can make if you have no oral rehydration salts for rehydration solution. They can help to prevent dehydration or they can be used as an early treatment for dehydration. Sugar and salt solution and coconut water with a pinch of salt are suitable to give patients at home or on the way to the health centre. If a fold of skin goes back slowly after you pinch it, the patient needs a solution made up with oral rehydration salts.

Sugar and salt solution

1. Use an empty clean soft drink bottle with '330 ml' written on the side. Use a clean metal top of the bottle.
2. Pour three full bottles of water into a bowl.
3. Use water from a safe supply, such as a protected well, protected rainwater or tap water. If you use water from a river this should be boiled and cooled if possible.
4. Use the bottle top to measure the amount of sugar and salt. Put 10 full bottletops of sugar and one flattened bottle top of salt into the water.
5. Mix the water until the sugar and salt dissolve. The solution is now ready to drink.
6. You may prefer to measure the water using a cup. Most cups contain about 200 ml. Put five cups of water into a bowl. You can measure the sugar and salt with your hand. Take one scoop of sugar in your hand but do not use your little finger (Picture 56). Pinch the salt with two fingers and your thumb (Picture 57).

Coconut water with a pinch of salt

Fresh coconut water does not need to be boiled. Coconut water with a pinch of salt is suitable for patients to use at home.
1. Take one young (green) coconut. Cut off the top.
2. Add one pinch of salt with two fingers and your thumb (see Picture 58) to the fluid inside the coconut.
3. Mix the coconut water by shaking it a little. The coconut water is now ready to drink.

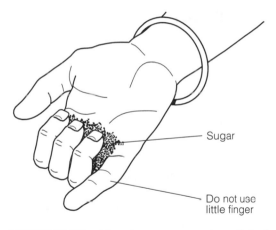

PICTURE 56 *How to measure a handful of sugar without using the little finger*

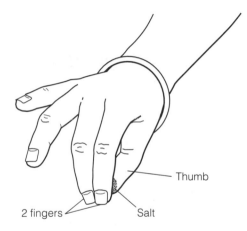

PICTURE 57 *How to measure a 2-fingered pinch of salt*

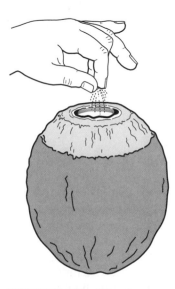

PICTURE 58 *How to measure a 2-fingered pinch of salt into a young coconut*

APPENDIX 13   Polio

Polio is also called poliomyelitis. Polio is a virus infection which is passed on in faeces.

Prevention

Polio infection is prevented by:
- vaccination
- good hygiene.

Polio vaccinations are given by mouth at birth, 6 weeks, 10 weeks, 14 weeks, and two more times between the age of 1 year and 5 years.

Signs and symptoms

1. Polio illness is usually very mild. The patient may have a sore throat, fever, headache and feel nauseated.
2. Sometimes, after 2 days, the patient has a more severe fever and has difficulty moving his leg or rarely his arm.
3. After 3 or 4 days, polio causes weakness which is worse on one side than the other. The muscles become painful and floppy. In a few weeks, the muscles become small. The muscles may become less weak over the next weeks or months.
4. The patient may not be able to breathe because the breathing muscles are weak and he could die.
5. To prevent these severe problems:
    - Make sure that children are given the polio vaccine, even if they are slightly unwell.
    - Teach people to follow the six rules of good nutrition.
    - Only give injections when there is no other suitable treatment.
6. If a patient develops muscle weakness 3 or 4 days after a fever and has painful muscles, treat him for acute polio.

Treatment of acute polio

1. Rest in bed until there has been no fever for 5 days.
2. Do not give any injections.
3. Give paracetamol for pain.
4. Move the patient's feet so thay are at right angles to the legs and slightly bend the knees. Support the knees from behind using a pillow. The hips and back should lie flat. The arms should be slightly bent.

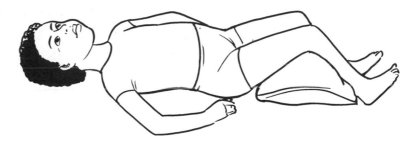

PICTURE 59   *Position for acute polio treatment*

5. Ask the patient to blow out a candle or match. If he cannot blow out the candle or match, he has difficult breathing. If he has difficult breathing, use a tube to suck away fluids from the back of the throat. Put in a nasogastric tube to give liquid food.

Treatment of polio after the fever and pain have gone

1. Move the muscles and joints several times each day. This will prevent the legs (or arms) from becoming bent forever.
2. Help the patient to stay active and independent. Walking aids or wheeled boards or chairs are helpful.
3. Tell the patient that there may be improvement in their movements for up to 18 months. It is important for someone to help them to move their joints regularly.
4. Some children will need help for several years to allow them to be as active and independent as possible.
5. The child should still be given all the usual vaccinations.

When not to diagnose polio

It can be easy to confuse polio with other illnesses that cause similar symptoms. Remember that polio does not cause problems with the feeling in the legs or arms.
If a patient has weakness:

- Look on the patient's skin for a tick. If you find a tick cover it with vaseline or oil. Wait for the tick to fall off. This may take 2 hours. Do not pull the tick off.
- Look for bite marks. The patient may have rabies.

If many people have weakness:

- Find out what they have eaten. Toxins in food can cause weakness. Botulin toxin, bitter cassava or grass pea poisoning are common.

APPENDIX 14　How to treat a woman with pain in the lower abdomen or unusual discharge from the private parts

Problem　　　　　　　　　　　　　　　　　　　　　　**Treatment**

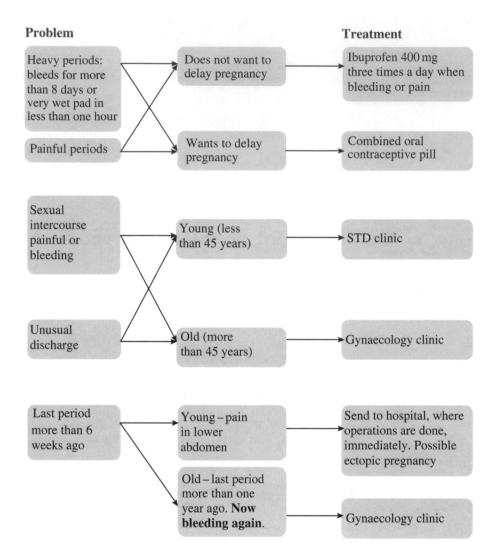

Problem		Treatment
Heavy periods: bleeds for more than 8 days or very wet pad in less than one hour	Does not want to delay pregnancy	Ibuprofen 400 mg three times a day when bleeding or pain
Painful periods	Wants to delay pregnancy	Combined oral contraceptive pill
Sexual intercourse painful or bleeding	Young (less than 45 years)	STD clinic
Unusual discharge	Old (more than 45 years)	Gynaecology clinic
Last period more than 6 weeks ago	Young – pain in lower abdomen	Send to hospital, where operations are done, immediately. Possible ectopic pregnancy
	Old – last period more than one year ago. **Now bleeding again**.	Gynaecology clinic

APPENDIX 15   How to treat obstetric problems

History	Examination	Diagnosis and treatment
Vomited four times or more today (may be early pregnancy)	This is a general danger sign ⟶	Treat for a very severe febrile disease. Do not give chloramphenicol. **Send to hospital immediately.**
Vomited fewer than four times today (may be early pregnancy)	Examine urine with microscope ⟶	If urinary tract infection give amoxicillin 250 mg three times a day for 5 days. If no urinary tract infection, she has **vomiting in early pregnancy.**
Severe pain in lower abdomen	Early pregnancy ⟶	Possible ectopic pregnancy. **Send to hospital immediately.** Give oral rehydration solution if has shock or peritonitis.
	Late pregnancy ⟶	If regular intermittent pain **send to hospital if labour** continues for more than 24 hours. If constant pain possible **ruptured uterus.** Often dizzy. Give oral rehydration solution. **Send to hospital immediately.**
Bleeding from private parts	Before 6 months ⟶	**Abortion or threatened abortion.** If has fever, give benzylpenicillin 2 million IU. If has more than small amount of blood **send her to hospital.** If no fever, small amount of blood: tell her to rest.
	After 6 months ⟶	**Antepartum haemorrhage. Send to hospital immediately.** Give oral rehydration solution 5 ml each minute.
	After birth ⟶	**Postpartum haemorrhage.** Pass urine, breastfeed, give ergometrine, oral rehydration solution, press uterus with both hands. If bleeding continues **take to hospital.**

227

APPENDIX 15 How to treat obstetric problems *Continued*

History	Examination	Diagnosis and treatment
Something hanging from private parts	**Prolapsed umbilical cord**	Push back if still has a pulse. Put bottom higher than head. **Send to hospital immediately.**
Convulsions	If still having a convulsion	Diazepam 10 mg rectally. Put on side. Magnesium sulphate 5 g in each leg. **Send to hospital immediately.**
	Convulsion has stopped	Magnesium sulphate 5 g in each leg. **Send to hospital immediately.**
Tired or palpitations	Pale conjunctivae → Measure haemoglobin	If less than 7 g/dl send to hospital for transfusion. If 7 g/dl to 10 g/dl give first line antimalarial if has fever. Mebendazole if has large number of hookworm eggs in faeces (not in first 3 months of pregnancy), Ferrous sulphate 200 mg three times a day for 3 months or more.

APPENDIX 16   Diabetes

A person with diabetes is not able to take sugar out of the blood. Patients with diabetes may not have enough insulin. There are two types of diabetes:

- Type 1 diabetes, also called insulin-dependent diabetes. Type 1 diabetes usually affects children and young adults. Patients with type 1 diabetes have to inject insulin.
- Type 2 diabetes, also called non-insulin-dependent diabetes. Type 2 diabetes usually affects older adults. Type 2 diabetes is treated by eating a special diet and often with tablets.

Most people with diabetes have type 2 diabetes. Very few patients have type 1 diabetes.

Signs and symptoms

1. Feeling thirsty all the time. Passing large amounts of urine. The patient may also lose weight.
2. Frequent skin infections and ulcers, especially if an ulcer is no better 2 weeks after treatment.
3. If the patient has two of the following problems:
   - weight loss
   - becomes tired easily with no obvious reason
   - poor eyesight
   - a yeast infection of the skin or oral candida.

Send a patient with any of these symptoms to hospital. Send patients who have diabetes to hospital immediately if they have a skin ulcer.

Patients with type 1 diabetes will become very ill if they do not use insulin, and will die at a young age if insulin is not available. Patients with type 1 diabetes sometimes become very ill with diabetic ketoacidosis.

Both type 1 and type 2 diabetes damage the blood vessels. Damaged blood vessels cause many problems:

- blindness
- myocardial infarction
- cerebrovascular incident
- kidney damage
- gangrene (dead toes or feet)
- nerve damage.

Treatment

1. Teach the patient to eat a mixed diet and to avoid sugar foods.
2. Teach the patient to eat more food before working hard or exercising.

3. Patients with type 1 diabetes need to inject themselves with insulin every day. The patient gives himself injections into the fat underneath the skin.
4. Other diabetes patients may take tablets to help the body take sugar out of the blood.
5. If a patient who uses injections or tablets feels light-headed, sweats or acts strangely, put some sugar into her mouth. Give her some carbohydrate food as soon as possible.
6. Teach the patient to eat more frequently when she is ill. Tell the patient to drink carbohydrate drinks regularly until she is well again. Thin maize porridge is an example of a carbohydrate drink. She should continue to take her tablets or to give herself injections as normal.
7. Advise all patients not to smoke.
8. Advise all patients to take regular exercise.

When to send patients to hospital immediately

Send a diabetes patient to hospital:

- If she is unconscious or moves less than usual when awake, even after putting sugar into her mouth

Low blood sugar will cause a patient to become unconscious. Low blood sugar can be caused by injecting too much insulin, or not eating enough food. Too much sugar in the blood may also cause a patient to become unconscious.

Before sending her to hospital, treat for very severe febrile disease. Give 50 ml of milk or sugar water through a nasogastric tube. Next, give oral rehydration solution, 5 ml each minute on the way to hospital. This is the correct treatment for both low blood sugar and diabetic ketoacidosis.

If a patient with diabetes is ill and her breath smells sweet, give her an injection of six units of insulin if possible. Give her oral rehydration solution, 5 ml each minute, on the way to the hospital.

APPENDIX 17   How to interpret urine results

White blood cells

White blood cells in the urine often mean that the patient has a urinary tract infection.

Red blood cells

Red blood cells in the urine can be caused by:

- Blood from inside a woman's uterus if she is having her period.
- A kidney stone if the patient has severe pain in area 3 or area 9 of the abdomen. (See Lesson 8.)
- A urinary tract infection. There will also be a lot of white blood cells in the urine.
- Schistosomiasis. There will also be schistosomiasis eggs in the settled urine. If you think a patient may have schistosomiasis, collect his urine between 12 noon and 2 pm. Allow the urine to settle for about 2 hours. Next, examine the urine with a microscope, and look for the *Schistosoma haematobium* eggs.
- Nephritis, which is a disease of the kidneys.

Nothing

If nothing is found in the urine the patient may have:

- Sexually transmitted disease (STD) – send the patient to the STD clinic.
- Irritation of the urethra – this is sometimes caused when a woman has sexual intercourse when the vagina is not lubricated. She will also pass urine frequently. Advise her to drink plenty of water.
- Threadworms – if the patient is a girl who complains that her private parts or anus itches she may have threadworms. Boys and adults also get this problem. Treat with mebendazole 100 mg two times a day for 3 days. Advise patients to wash their hands with water and soap or ash, especially before they eat and after they use the latrine. Treat the whole family if possible.

APPENDIX 18 How to treat a patient with abdominal pain or with blood in the faeces

Questions

1. Do you have any problems when you pass urine?
2. Are your bowels all right?
3. When was your last normal menstrual period? Does your pain come at the same time as your period? Do you feel pain when you have sexual intercourse?
4. Show me where you feel the pain.
5. What type of pain do you feel? Is the pain constant or intermittent?
6. Is there anyone else at home who has the same symptoms that you have?

If passed loose or watery faeces three times or more this morning. Look at diarrhoea chart (Appendix 10)

Examination

1. Look for fever, anaemia and jaundice.
2. Look for swellings and tenderness.
If there is severe abdominal pain or blood in the faeces:
3. Look for guarding or rebound tenderness.

Examination normal:
1. Pain passing urine or passing urine frequently. **Send others to have urine examined.** Give amoxicillin if pregnant. **Send others to have urine examined.** Not able to pass urine. In pain. **Send to hospital immediately.**
2. Last normal period more than 6 weeks ago, **and** abdominal pain. **Send to hospital immediately.**
3. Gastroenteritis or food poisoning **and no** dehydration **and** passed faeces less than six times today. Home treatment for diarrhoea.

Examination findings and diagnosis

Fever:
In malaria areas test for malaria or treat with first-line malaria treatment.

Anaemia: Send immediately to hospital if has fast breathing or swollen legs.

Jaundice: Send immediately to hospital.

Swellings:
1. Woman with large abdominal swelling and pain in area 6 or low back. This is labour if the pains are regular.
2. Patient with swelling near centre of abdomen and pain. This may be intussusception.
3. Patient with painful swelling near private parts. This may be an incarcerated hernia.
4. Patient with swollen abdomen and pain. This may be a volvulus.
5. Rectal prolapse. Use vegetable oil. Push back into anus.

Tenderness:
In area 12 may be a peptic ulcer or gastritis.
In area 3 or 9 may be a kidney infection.
In area 5, 6 or 7 may be pelvic inflammatory disease or a urinary tract infection.
In area 10 or 11 may be hepatitis.

Guarding or rebound tenderness. The patient has peritonitis. Peritonitis may be caused by appendicitis, a perforated gastric ulcer, intussusception, an incarcerated hernia, an ectopic pregnancy, pelvic inflammatory disease, typhoid or a volvulus.

Send to hospital

If no better 2 days after starting first or second-line malaria treatment.

If labour lasts more than one day and one night or woman has been pushing for more than 2 hours.

Any patient who may have an intussusception, incarcerated hernia, a volvulus or a rectal prolapse.

Pain in area 12 for 2 weeks or more.

All patients with fever and pain in area 3 or 9.

If there is pain in area 5, 6 or 7 and the pain is made worse by sexual intercourse send to the sexually transmitted disease clinic with partner.

If there is pain in area 10 or 11 **and** fever or jaundice send to hospital immediately.

All patients with peritonitis. If the patient may have an ectopic pregnancy give her 5 ml of oral rehydration salts solution every minute.

APPENDIX 19 How to diagnose the cause of back pain

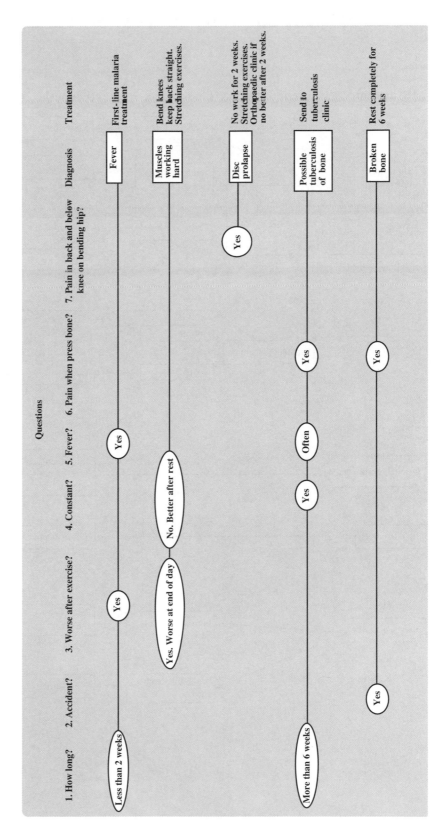

APPENDIX 20   How to treat an ear problem

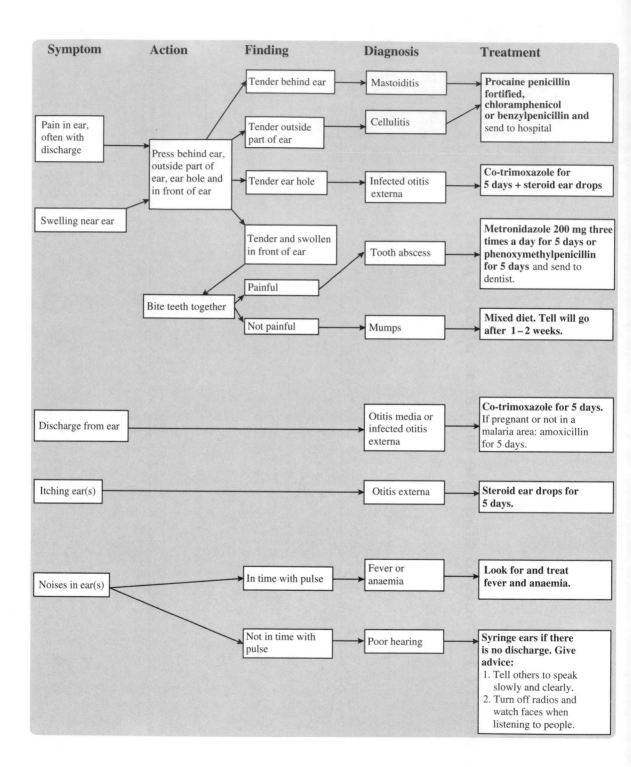

Symptom	Action	Finding	Diagnosis	Treatment
Pain in ear, often with discharge	Press behind ear, outside part of ear, ear hole and in front of ear	Tender behind ear	Mastoiditis	**Procaine penicillin fortified, chloramphenicol or benzylpenicillin and** send to hospital
		Tender outside part of ear	Cellulitis	
		Tender ear hole	Infected otitis externa	**Co-trimoxazole for 5 days + steroid ear drops**
Swelling near ear		Tender and swollen in front of ear	Tooth abscess	**Metronidazole 200 mg three times a day for 5 days or phenoxymethylpenicillin for 5 days and send to** dentist.
	Bite teeth together	Painful		
		Not painful	Mumps	**Mixed diet. Tell will go after 1–2 weeks.**
Discharge from ear			Otitis media or infected otitis externa	**Co-trimoxazole for 5 days.** If pregnant or not in a malaria area: amoxicillin for 5 days.
Itching ear(s)			Otitis externa	**Steroid ear drops for 5 days.**
Noises in ear(s)		In time with pulse	Fever or anaemia	**Look for and treat fever and anaemia.**
		Not in time with pulse	Poor hearing	**Syringe ears if there is no discharge. Give advice:** 1. Tell others to speak slowly and clearly. 2. Turn off radios and watch faces when listening to people.

APPENDIX 21 How to treat an eye problem

| Column 1
Type of
problem | Column 2
Look for main
symptoms
and signs | Column 3
Group
diagnosis | Column 4
Look for other
symptoms
and signs | Column 5
Diagnosis and treatment |

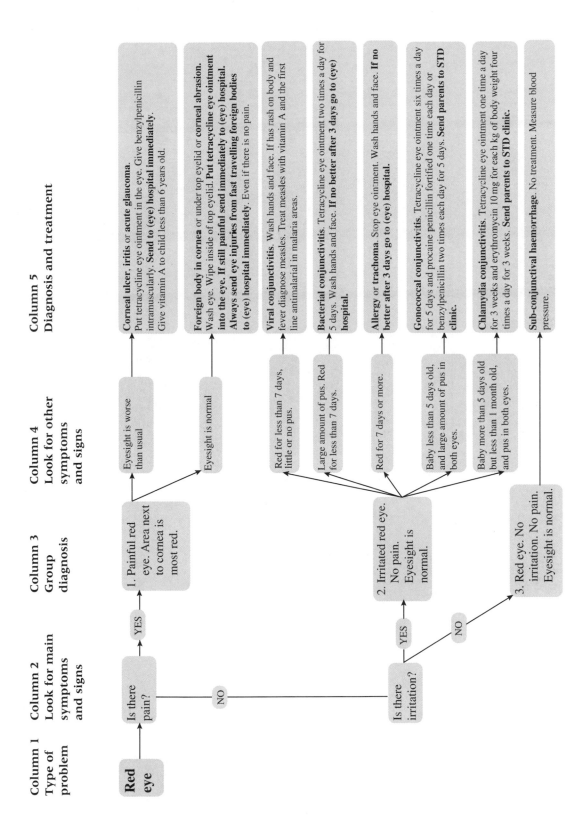

Corneal ulcer, iritis or **acute glaucoma.**
Put tetracycline eye ointment in the eye. Give benzylpenicillin
intramuscularly. **Send to (eye) hospital immediately.**
Give vitamin A to child less than 6 years old.

Foreign body in cornea or under top eyelid or **corneal abrasion.**
Wash eye. Wipe inside of top eyelid. **Put tetracycline eye ointment
into the eye. If still painful send immediately to (eye) hospital.
Always send eye injuries from fast travelling foreign bodies
to (eye) hospital immediately.** Even if there is no pain.

Viral conjunctivitis. Wash hands and face. If has rash on body and
fever diagnose measles. Treat measles with vitamin A and the first
line antimalarial in malaria areas.

Bacterial conjunctivitis. Tetracycline eye ointment two times a day for
5 days. Wash hands and face. **If no better after 3 days go to (eye)
hospital.**

Allergy or trachoma. Stop eye ointment. Wash hands and face. **If no
better after 3 days go to (eye) hospital.**

Gonococcal conjunctivitis. Tetracycline eye ointment six times a day
for 5 days and procaine penicillin fortified one time each day or
benzylpenicillin two times each day for 5 days. **Send parents to STD
clinic.**

Chlamydia conjunctivitis. Tetracycline eye ointment one time a day
for 3 weeks and erythromycin 10mg for each kg of body weight four
times a day for 3 weeks. **Send parents to STD clinic.**

Sub-conjunctival haemorrhage. No treatment. Measure blood
pressure.

Column 1
Type of problem

Column 2
Look for main symptoms and signs

Column 3
Group diagnosis

Column 4
Look for other symptoms and signs

Column 5
Diagnosis and treatment

Poor eyesight. Eye *not* red.

Can you make the eyesight better using multiple pin hole occluder? — YES → **4. Needs glasses or hand lens.** → Send to eye clinic for glasses.

NO ↓

Child's eyes look in different directions. — YES → **5. Possibly cross-eyed.** → Light reflection test. → **Cross-eyed. Send to eye clinic.**

NO ↓

Is the eyesight poor only after sunset? — YES → **6. Poor eyesight at night.** → There are dry areas on the cornea. → **Lack of vitamin A.** Give vitamin A three times in 2 weeks. Teach 6 rules of good nutrition.

NO → **7. Poor eyesight day and night.**

— YES → The pupil is not black. → **Cataract. Send to eye clinic.**

— YES → The cornea is not clear. → **Corneal scar** from **trachoma** or **onchocerciasis** . **If there is pain or irritation** put tetracycline eye ointment in the eye and **send to (eye) hospital immediately.** If in an onchocerciasis area treat with ivermectin 6 mg each year.

— YES → It is difficult to see things to the side. → **Chronic glaucoma. Send to eye clinic.**

Swelling next to the eye.

Is the patient unwell with fever? — YES → Fever, pain, swelling of top and bottom eyelids. Red eye. → **Orbital cellulitis.** Tetracycline eye ointment. Benzylpenicillin. **Send to hospital immediately**

NO ↓

Is there a painful swelling underneath eye next to the nose? — YES → Pain is worse when you press the swelling and pus comes into the eye. → **Acute dacrocystitis.** Phenoxymethylpenicillin three times a day for 5 days. 125 mg if 10 to 19 kg. 250 mg if 20 to 40 kg. 500 mg if more than 40 kg. Press swelling three times a day. **Go to eye clinic if no better after treatment**

NO ↓

Is there swelling in one eyelid? — YES → Swelling is near to the eyelashes. Swelling is painful when you touch it. → **Stye** or infected **meibomian cyst.** Tetracycline eye ointment two times a day for 5 days. **Go to eye clinic if no better after treatment**

APPENDIX 22 Prescriber's checklists

Health centre tutorials

Work with each student in a primary health centre after each lesson. Watch the student as he does each thing that he has learned. Watch him do the following things:

- take a history
- examine patients
- write a summary of what he has found
- use the chart which summarises how to treat the problem (if there is a chart)
- decide what the diagnosis is
- decide what medicine to give to the patient
- give advice to the patient
- communicate with the patient.

Use the trainer's copy of the Prescriber's checklist to remind you what the student should have learnt in the last lesson. After the student has seen each patient, use the student's copy to write down what you observed (see p. 243). Make sure that the patient was given the correct treatment and advice.

Trainer's copy

After lesson	1	2	3	4	5	6
			Skills and knowledge to look for			
How to take a patient's history	Knows the 4 *general danger signs*	Knows how to treat a patient who has a *general danger sign*	Takes the patient's history	Looks at the growth chart of all children less than 5 years old	If the patient has pain in the abdomen or blood in the faeces the student follows the advice on Appendix 18	Writes a summary of what she has found

Skills and knowledge to look for

After lesson	1	2	3	4	5	6
Communication	Uses a quiet place to talk	Uses simple language	Looks at patient's eyes	Tells patient about the problem, the treatment, and when to return	Gives only one medicine to use at home if possible	Asks patient how they will use their medicine
Lesson 1 Rational Prescribing	Uses curative medicines where possible	Gives patients the correct medicine. Gives no medicine if no medicine is needed	Gives correct dose for correct length of time	Gives generic medicine	Usually gives one medicine	Gives patient education or advice
Lesson 2 Chest problems	Does not give an antibiotic for upper respiratory tract infections	Knows the signs of respiratory distress. Gives patients with respiratory distress a rapid-acting bronchodilator, an injection of benzylpenicillin and sends him to hospital	Counts how many times the patient breathes in one minute. Knows what fast breathing is in all patients	Uses Appendix 1 and Appendix 2 to decide how to treat patients with a cough or difficult breathing	Teaches the mother home treatment for chest illnesses	Knows the correct treatment for a wheeze
Lesson 3 Fever, malaria convulsions and meningitis	Treats all children with a fever with the first-line malaria treatment in malaria areas	Tells patients to return if their fever is no better after 2 days	Takes the patient's history and looks for *general danger signs*	If a patient has a fever which is no better after the first-line malaria treatment the student looks for a cause for the fever. If there is no obvious cause he sends the patient to hospital or treats the patient with the second-line malaria treatment	Teaches mothers how to tepid sponge	Treats patients with a general danger sign correctly

Lesson 4 Malnutrition and anaemia	Looks at growth charts of all children under 5 years	Uses Appendix 6 to decide how to treat children with malnutrition or anaemia	There is a person at the health centre who teaches mothers the six rules of good nutrition	Looks for swelling of the legs if the growth line is flat or going down	Sends patients to nutrition clinic if growth line has gone down on the two most recent weighings	Treats moderate anaemia correctly
Lesson 5 Skin problems	Does not treat scabies with antibiotics. He may use an antibiotic if there is a large area of impetigo	Thinks of measles if a patient has a fever *and* a rash all over his body. The rash does *not* itch. Diagnoses measles if the patient also has red eyes *or* a cough *or* fluid coming from the nose	Gives children with measles Vitamin A at the health centre	Does not treat patients with measles or chickenpox with antibiotics. Antibiotics may be used if the patient has a complication of measles, pneumonia for example	Gives patients with skin ulcers tetanus vaccination if needed	Stops medicines which may have caused a reaction
Lesson 6 Diarrhoea	Uses Appendix 10 to decide how to treat patients with diarrhoea	Pinches the skin of all patients with diarrhoea. Teaches mothers to breast feed babies for 2 years	Teaches mothers home treatment if the skin goes back quickly after it is pinched	Treats diarrhoea with antibiotics *only if* the patient is a child, has malnutrition, dysentery, is very ill or is no better after 5 days	Gives oral rehydration salts (ORS) solution to patients who have been treated for dehydration. Shows how to prepare ORS solution	Sends patients who have passed very watery faeces six times or more to a cholera treatment centre after 4–6 hours of treatment with ORS solution
Lesson 7 Women's health problems	Treats heavy or painful periods with ibuprofen or the combined oral contraceptive pill	Measures the haemoglobin of pale pregnant women. Uses Appendix 6 to decide how to treat anaemia	Advises all pregnant women to eat a mixed diet. Gives all pregnant women ferrous sulphate and folic acid	Sends pregnant women with a blood pressure of 95 mmHg or more to hospital	Knows how to treat a woman who is having a post partum haemorrhage	If a woman's last normal period was more than 6 weeks ago, and the woman has severe lower

Skills and knowledge to look for

After lesson	1	2	3	4	5	6
						abdominal pain, the student immediately sends the woman to a hospital which does operations
Lesson 8 Abdominal problems	Knows how to look for peritonitis. Knows to send patients with peritonitis immediately to a hospital which does operations	Always examines abdomen if patient has abdominal pain or blood in the faeces	Uses Appendix 18 to decide how to treat a patient with abdominal pain or blood in the faeces	Does not give aspirin or ibuprofen to patients with abdominal pain	If a patient has a swelling near the centre of the abdomen and pain, sends patient immediately to a hospital where operations are done	If a patient has painful swelling near the private parts, sends the patient immediately to a hospital where operations are done
Lesson 9 Heart problems	Knows how to measure the blood pressure	Sends patients with an **average** blood pressure of 105 mmHg or higher to hospital	Gives four pieces of advice to patients with high blood pressure	Listens to the heart of all patients who have fast breathing but no fever	Sends patients with swollen ankles or crackles in both lungs, to hospital immediately	Treats patients with a possible myocardial infarction with aspirin 300mg

Lesson 10 Accidents emergencies, joints and backs	Sends patients to hospital if any of the five head injury questions are yes	Gives tetanus vaccination to patients with cuts or wounds if needed	Knows treatment for shock and anaphylaxis	Knows when to use antibiotics for burns and when to send burns patients to hospital	Looks for swelling, heat, tenderness and pain on bending the joint if a joint is painful. Sends patients with possible septic arthritis to hospital immediately	Uses Appendix 19 to diagnose the cause of back pain
Lesson 11 Psychiatric problems	Treats patients with a severe mental illness, *and* fever for a very severe febrile disease	Sends patients with a severe mental illness *and* fever, *or* a severe mental illness after a head injury, to hospital immediately	Knows the treatment for acute dystonia	Sends a patient with three or more symptoms of depression, or a patient who plans to kill himself, to see a psychiatric doctor or nurse	Looks for more important psychiatric problems if a patient has anxiety or depression	Counsels patients with anxiety or depression
Lesson 12 Tuberculosis and leprosy	Sends all patients with symptoms of tuberculosis to clinic	Stops tuberculosis medicines if the patient gets jaundice. Sends the patient to the next tuberculosis clinic	Stops tuberculosis medicines if the patient gets blisters in and around the mouth and eyes. Sends the patient to the next tuberculosis clinic	Sends all patients with symptoms or signs of leprosy to clinic	Treats reversal reactions and ENL reactions with paracetamol and tells patient to continue leprosy medicine	Knows what advice should and be given to leprosy patients (this is normally given in the leprosy clinic)

Skills and knowledge to look for

After lesson	1	2	3	4	5	6
Lesson 13 HIV disease	Knows which infections are made more common by HIV	Gives correct treatment for infections which are made more common by HIV	Tells patients with HIV to have all the normal vaccinations	Counsels patients before doing an HIV test	Teaches people how to avoid getting HIV	Sends all patients with symptoms of a sexually transmitted disease to the sexually transmitted disease clinic
Lesson 14 Ear, nose and throat problems	Treats patients with otitis media with co-trimoxazole in malaria areas. Treats pregnant women or patients in other areas with amoxicillin	Does not give antibiotics for viral tonsillitis	Advises patients with pain in the mouth to eat a mixed diet and to brush their teeth	Knows what the symptoms of diphtheria are. Knows how to treat diphtheria	Does not examine the throat of a patient who has a painful throat *and* is not able to drink. Treats possible epiglottitis with benzyl-penicillin and sends to hospital immediately	Measures the blood pressure of patients who have blood coming from the nose
Lesson 15 Eye problems	Uses Appendix 21 to decide how to treat eye problems	Treats the five types of conjunctivitis correctly	Advises patients with conjunctivitis to wash the eyes and hands often and not to use the same towel as others	Is able to examine eyes correctly	Treats night blindness with vitamin A. Treats children under 6 with corneal ulcers with vitamin A	If a patient has poor eyesight with no obvious cause the student looks for fever, anaemia, measures blood pressure and tests urine for sugar (in hospital)

Student's copy

Student: _____ Clinic: _____

After lesson	Does well		Areas to improve	
Chapter 2 How to take a patient's history				
Chapter 3 Communication				
Lesson 1 Rational prescribing				
Lesson 2 Chest problems				
Lesson 3 Fever, malaria convulsions and meningitis				
Lesson 4 Malnutrition and anaemia				
Lesson 5 Skin problems				
Lesson 6 Diarrhoea				

After lesson	Does well		Areas to improve	
Lesson 7 Women's health problems				
Lesson 8 Abdominal problems				
Lesson 9 Heart problems				
Lesson 10 Accidents, emergencies, joints and the back				
Lesson 11 Psychiatric problems				
Lesson 12 Tuberculosis and leprosy				
Lesson 13 HIV disease				
Lesson 14 Ear, nose and throat problems				
Lesson 15 Eye problems				

APPENDIX 23   List of medicines and their uses

Abbreviations:
×1/day = one time a day; ×2/day = two times a day; ×3/day – three times a day; ×4/day = four times a day
×1 = one time only
½ = one half; ¼ = one quarter
+ = and above
Tab = tablet

Medicine	Uses	Dose
Acetylsalicylic acid (ASA), (aspirin). Tab 300 mg.	Reduces pain. Do *not* use for abdominal pain. Aspirin is a symptomatic medicine.	*Age* *Dose* 1–2 years ¼ tab 3–6 years ½ tab 7–12 years 1 tab 13+ years 2 tab Take this dose no more than 4 times a day. Take after food.
Adrenaline: *see* epinephrine.		
Albendazole. Tab 200 mg or 400 mg.	Removes hookworm, round-worm, whipworm and threadworm. Do not give to pregnant women.	*Age* *Dose* 2–5 years 200 mg × 1 6 years or more 400 mg × 1
Aluminium hydroxide. Tab 500 mg.	For gastritis. If patient has pain in the upper abdomen for less than 2 weeks (area 12) *but does not have* guarding or rebound tenderness. If the pain continues for more than 2 weeks, go to hospital. He may have a peptic ulcer.	Chew one tablet each time he feels pain in the upper abdomen. Give 30 tablets.
Aminophylline. Tab 100 mg.	For patients with wheeze *without* signs of respiratory distress and *no* fast breathing.	*Age* *Dose* 0–11 months ¼ tab × 3/day 1–5 years ½ tab × 3/day 6+ years 1 tab × 3/day Give 5 days treatment.

Medicine	Uses	Dose
Amoxicillin. Tab 250 mg or 500 mg. Liquid 125 mg in 5 ml.	For pregnant women with a UTI or sinusitis. For pregnant women with a kidney infection. For pneumonia, bronchitis, otitis media, infected otitis externa or sinusitis (for children). **NOT** for tonsillitis.	250 mg × 3/day 500 mg × 3/day *Age* *Dose* 0–2 months 62.5 mg × 3/day 2–11 months 125 mg × 3/day 1–10 years 250 mg × 3/day 11 + years 500 mg × 3/day Give 5 days treatment.
Aspirin: *see* acetylsalicylic acid.		
Benzoic acid and salicylic acid (Whitfield ointment).	For a fungus infection of the skin.	Rub onto the affected area only × 1/day for many weeks. Use for at least 4 weeks. If no better after 4 weeks send the patient to the leprosy clinic. If the affected area is smaller after 4 weeks continue to use Whitfield ointment until the rash has gone completely, *and* for 1 more week.
Benzyl benzoate emulsion 25% (BBE). 100 ml (Dilute concentrate (90%) before use. Add one part of concentrate to three parts of clean warm water. Use within 4 weeks.)	For scabies. Treat whole family. Rub into every part of the body apart from the face and head. Do *not* wash for 24 hours. Put on again after 7 days.	One bottle of benzyl benzoate (25%) for two adults or children over the age of 5 (each bottle holds 100 ml). For children under the age of 2 years mix the benzyl benzoate with an equal amount of water. Give enough to treat the whole family, even if they have no symptoms.
Chloramphenicol. 1000 mg powder in vial. Add 5 ml sterile water. Shake until clear.	For severe infections that cause a *general danger sign*. For epiglottitis mastoiditis or cellulitis near the ear. Give intramuscularly.	40 mg (0.2 ml) for each kg one time. Do not give more than 1000 mg (5.6 ml). Repeat after 12 hours if the patient is not able to get to the hospital. Do not give for longer than 5 days.

Medicine	Uses	Dose
Chloroquine phosphate. Tab 150 mg (base) or liquid 50 mg (base) in each 5 ml.	For malaria. If the patient has a fever in a malaria area and you cannot test for malaria.	Three days of treatment: Day 1: 10 mg/kg × 1 Day 2: 10 mg/kg × 1 Day 3: 5 mg/kg × 1 For an adult who weighs 45.5 kg or more do not give more than 600 mg/ 600 mg/300 mg (4/4/2 tablets).
Chloroquine phosphate injection 40 mg in each 1 ml.	For malaria if the patient has a *general danger sign*. Give intramuscularly.	3.5 mg for each kg one time. Do not give more than 200 mg for an adult. Repeat after 8 hours if the patient is still vomiting. Give tablets when the patient is no longer vomiting.
Co-trimoxazole. Tab 480 mg, or liquid 240 mg in each 5 ml. (5 ml = ½ Tab) Note: 480 mg of co-trimoxazole consists of sulphamethoxazole 400 mg and trimethoprim 80 mg.	For pneumonia, bronchitis cellulitis, abscess, large areas of impetigo, acute dacrocystitis, dysentery, otitis media, infected otitis externa or sinusitis. For orchitis if *no* pain on passing urine or discharge from the penis. Also for UTI *after* the urine has been examined under a microscope. For osteomyelitis or a sickle-cell crisis (and septic arthritis if will not be at hospital within 6 hours).	*Age* *Dose* 0–6 months 2.5 ml (½ tea-spoon) × 2/day *or* ¼ tab × 2/day 7 months– ½ tab × 2/day 5 years 6–12 years 1 tab × 2/day 13+ years 2 tab × 2/day Give 5 days treatment. Two times the normal dose.
Combined oral contraceptive. Many types.	To delay pregnancy. To treat heavy periods or painful periods *if* does *not* want to become pregnant at present.	*Most pills:* One pill every day. *Some pills:* One pill every day for 21 days and do not take a pill for 7 days. Next, start again on the 29th day. All pills may be used for several years.
Diazepam. Rectal solution. 5 mg or 10 mg in a rectal tube.	When the patient is having a convulsion. For large broken bones.	*Age* *Dose* Less than 1 year 2.5 mg 1–3 years 5 mg 4 years or more 10 mg

Medicine	Uses	Dose
Diazepam (continued)		Give one more dose if still convulsing 5 minutes after first dose.

Epinephrine (adrenaline). Injection 1 in 1000.	If patient has signs of respiratory distress. Also give benzylpenicillin, chloramphenicol or procaine penicillin and send to hospital. *Inject sub-cutaneously* (under the skin).
	
	For anaphylaxis: *Inject intramuscularly.*
		Age *Dose*
		0–11 months 0.1 ml
		
		1–4 years 0.25 ml
		             (¼ vial)
		
		5 + years 0.5 ml
		             (½ vial)
		
		Repeat if still unconscious or unwell 10 minutes after first injection.

Ergometrine. Injection 0.5 mg for each ml (1 ml in vial). Store in a cool place, preferably a fridge.	Prevents or treats postpartum haemorrhage. For women who have just given birth. *After all the babies have been born.*	0.5 mg × 1 into a muscle to prevent postpartum haemorrhage. 0.5 mg × 1 into a vein (or muscle) to treat postpartum haemorrhage.
Erythromycin. Tab 250 mg.	For chlamydia conjunctitivitis.	10 mg for each kg × 3/day for 21 days.
Fansidar: *see* pyrimethamine + sulfadoxine.		
Ferrous sulphate. Tab 200 mg (60 mg of iron) or ferrous sulphate 200 mg with folic acid 0.25 mg.	For anaemia after its causes have been treated (treat for malaria and hookworm and advise about a mixed diet first). All pregnant women.	*Weight* *Dose* 0–15 kg ¼ tab × 2/day 16–29 kg ½ tab × 2/day 30–44 kg 1 tab × 2/day 45 + kg 1 tab × 3/day Treat for at least 3 months. 1 tab every day for the whole pregnancy.
Folic acid. Tab 0.4 mg, Tab 1 mg or Tab 5 mg.	All pregnant women. For sickle cell disease: treats and prevents anaemia.	0.4 mg every day for the whole pregnancy. 5 mg every day, forever.
Gentian violet: *see* methylrosanilinium chloride.		

Medicine	Uses	Dose
Ibuprofen. Tab 200 mg or Tab 400 mg.	For painful periods and heavy periods. For kidney stones.	400 mg × 3/day only when the period starts and for 3–5 days. 600 mg × 3/day when there is pain. Stop ibuprofen if has pain in upper abdomen.
Lidocaine hydrochloride. (lignocaine). Injection 1% or 2%.	Inject into the muscle around a new wound before cleaning and stitching it. Make sure that the needle is not in a vein by pulling back the plunger on the syringe before injecting.	Not more than 20 ml of 1%. Not more than 10 ml of 2%.
Magnesium sulphate. Injection.	For eclampsia. If a pregnant woman has a convulsion.	5 g intramuscularly into *each* leg. After 4 hours give 2.5 g into *each* leg.
Mebendazole. Tab 100 mg.	Removes hookworm, round-worm, whipworm and threadworm. *Not* for women in the first 3 months of pregnancy.	*Age* *Dose* 1 + year 100 mg × 2/day Give treatment for 3 days.
Methylrosanilinium chloride (Gentian violet) crystals 5 g (one heaped teaspoon) to be dissolved in 1 litre of water. Strain mixture or carefully pour into a new bottle to remove any sediment.	For impetigo if less than 10 cm wide. For oral candida.	Paint one time a day for 5 days. Rinse mouth two times a day for 7 days.
Metronidazole. Tab 200 mg or 250 mg.	For a tooth abscess. Send the patient to the dentist.	200 mg or 250 mg × 3/day for 5 days. It is dangerous to drink alcohol when using metronidazole.
Multivitamins. Tab.	These are *not* useful to treat or prevent malnutrition. Teach patients how to grow and eat a mixed diet.	1 tab × 1/day for 5 days.

Medicine	Uses	Dose
Multivitamins (continued)	If a patient does not need any medicine but they insist that you give them a medicine, give them multivitamins. Multivitamins will not harm the patient.	
Nalidixic acid. Tab 500 mg.	Second-line treatment for dysentery.	*Age* *Dose* 2–11 months ¼ × 4/day 1–4 years ½ × 4/day 5–12 years 1 × 4/day 13 + years 2 × 4/day Give treatment for 5 days.
Normal saline.	For cleaning wounds and ulcers.	On the first visit squirt normal saline or clean water quickly at the ulcer. Do this until all the dirt has been removed. On other visits clean *very gently* using a sterile swab or cloth dipped in normal saline to avoid damaging the healing red skin.
Oral rehydration salts (ORS). One packet to be dissolved in 1 litre of water (3 × 330 ml soft drink bottles).	To treat dehydration. To prevent dehydration after treating dehydration. To treat shock on the way to the hospital.	See Appendix 10: How to treat diarrhoea. To prevent dehydration tell patients to drink the fluids they usually drink and *extra* fluid. Give extra fluid after each loose faeces: *Age* *Extra* *Take home* *fluid* 0–2 years 100 ml 2 packets 2–9 years 200 ml 2 packets 10 + years 400 ml 4 packets Tell the patient that ORS will not stop the diarrhoea. Give ORS which has been made up. Tell her to drink 5 ml every minute.

Medicine	Uses	Dose
Paracetamol. Tab 500 mg.	Reduces pain. Paracetamol is a symptomatic medicine.	*Age* *Dose* 0–5 years ¼ tab × 4/day 6–12 years ½ tab × 4/day 13+ years 1 or 2 tab × 4/day *Do not use more than these doses.* Give enough tablets for 2 days treatment.
	For osteoarthritis or rheumatoid arthritis.	Give 8 tablets a day for osteoarthritis and rheumatoid arthritis.
Penicillin Benzylpenicillin (Crystalline penicillin or 'X pen'). Injection 5 million IU (3000 mg) in a vial. 1 million IU = 600 mg.	For severe infections that cause a *general danger sign*. Send patient to hospital immediately: For a painful red eye if the eyesight is worse than usual. For a sickle-cell crisis.	0.1 million IU (60 mg) for each kg of body weight × 1 (or 4 times a day if the patient is not able to get to the hospital immediately). Do not give more than 2 million IU. Inject into a muscle.
Procaine penicillin fortified (PPF). Injection 4 million IU (4000 mg) in a vial. 1 million IU = 1000 mg.	For infections which need a large dose of antibiotic. For cellulitis or mastoiditis. Send to hospital immediately. For gonococcal conjunctivitis (also give tetracycline eye ointment).	0.1 million IU (100 mg) for each kg of body weight one time every day for 5 days. Do not give more than 1.2 million IU. Inject intramuscularly.
Phenoxymethylpenicillin (Pen V). Tab 250 mg.	For tonsillitis, acute dacrocystitis, cellulitis, pneumonia, a tooth abscess or a large area of impetigo (greater than 10 cm across).	*Weight* *Dose* 10–19 kg 125 mg × 3/day 20–39 kg 250 mg × 3/day 40 kg or more 500 mg × 3/day Give 5 days treatment.
Polyvidone iodine 10%. (povidone iodine).	For cleaning wounds and ulcers.	On the first visit use a syringe to push normal saline or clean water quickly at the ulcer until all the dirt has been removed. Then put polyvidone iodine on the wound. On other

Medicine	Uses	Dose
Polyvidone iodine (continued)		visits clean *very gently* using a sterile swab or cloth dipped in polyvidone iodine to avoid damaging the healing red skin.
Pyrimethamine 25 mg + sulfadoxine 500 mg Tab. (Fansidar)	For malaria. If the patient has a fever in a malaria area and you cannot test for malaria.	*Age* *Dose* less than 4 years ½ tab × 1 4–6 years 1 tab × 1 7–9 years 1½ tab × 1 10–14 years 2 tab × 1 15+ years 3 tab × 1 Give only one dose.
Quinine. Tab 300 mg (sometimes 200 mg).	For malaria which is resistant to the first-line antimalarial in your country: • If a fever is no better after using chloroquine or Fansidar. • If a fever returns before 2 weeks have passed *and* there is no obvious cause for the fever. If the patient has a *general danger sign* or is less than 5 years old send him to hospital.	10 mg for each kg × 3/day. Do not give more than 600 mg × 3/day. Give 7 days treatment.
Quinine. Injection 150 mg in each 1 ml or 300 mg in each 1 ml.	For malaria if the patient has a *general danger sign*. Give quinine intramuscularly.	10 mg for each kg one time. Do not give more than 600 mg for an adult. Repeat after 8 hours if the patient is still vomiting. Give tablets when the patient is no longer vomiting.
Retinol (vitamin A). Tab (capsules) 25,000 IU, 50,000 IU, 100,000 IU, 200,000 IU.	For night blindness, Bitot's spots, patients under 6 years old with a corneal ulcer, severe malnutrition and measles.	*Age* *Dose* 0–1 year 100,000 IU 3 times 1+ years 200,000 IU 3 times Give the first dose immediately. Give the second dose on the following day or after finishing an antimalarial.

Medicine	Uses	Dose
Retinol (continued)		Give the third dose 2 weeks later. Also advise about a mixed diet.
Salbutamol. Tab 2 mg or 4 mg.	For wheeze if there are *no* signs of respiratory distress and does *not* have fast breathing.	*Age* *Dose* Less than 1 mg×3/day 1 year 1–4 years 2 mg×3/day 5+years 4 mg×3/day Give 5 days treatment.
Salbutamol. Metered dose inhaler.	For patients with signs of respiratory distress. Also give benzylpenicillin and send to hospital.	Through a spacer (a plastic bottle). Shake before pressing Press 1 time for each time the patient breathes 5 times. Repeat 10 times.
Tetracycline. Tab 250 mg.	For sinusitis if patient is 13 years or more and *not* pregnant. (Also used in the treatment of cholera. The dose is different.)	250 mg×3/day. Give 5 days treatment.
Tetracycline eye ointment. 4 g tube 1%.	For *conjunctivitis caused by bacteria.*	×2/day for 5 days.
	For *trachoma.*	×3/day for 1 week then ×2/day for 5 more weeks.
	For *conjunctivitis caused by chlamydia* (child older than 5 days but less than 1 month), together with erythromycin.	×1/day for 3 weeks.
	For *conjunctivitis caused by gonococcus* (child less than 5 days old) together with procaine penicillin fortified.	6 times a day for 5 days.
	For a *corneal ulcer.*	×1 also give an injection of Benzylpenicillin then send to hospital.
Vitamin A: *see* retinol.		
Whitfield Ointment: *see* benzoic acid and salicylic acid.		

Glossary

abscess: a swelling under the skin filled with *pus*.

abdomen: the part of the body that contains the stomach, *bowel* and many other organs.

abortion: the unborn baby dies inside the *uterus* before the woman has been pregnant for 6 months.

allergy: a reaction to medicine, food or an insect bite. The reaction is often sneezing, an itchy rash, or difficult breathing. Allergies can be very dangerous.

antibiotic: medicine used to fight *bacteria*.

antibodies: the weapons that the body uses to fight *infection*.

anus: the hole at the end of the *bowel* where *faeces* leave the body.

artery: a tube which carries blood away from the heart. There is a *pulse* when you touch an artery.

bacteria: small germs which can cause infectious illness. *Antibiotics* fight bacteria.

birth: the time when a baby comes out of the *uterus*.

bladder: the bag inside the *abdomen* that stores *urine*.

bowel: intestine.

cancer: a *disease* that spreads inside the body and may cause death.

cervix: the neck or opening of the *uterus* inside the *vagina*.

chest indrawing: the skin is pulled in when the patient breathes in.

cholera: an illness in which the patient passes a large amount of very watery *faeces*.

clinic: a place where trained health workers see patients with a special type of problem, often in a hospital.

condom: a narrow rubber sheath that a man wears on his penis during *sexual intercourse*. Condoms prevent sexually transmitted diseases, including HIV, and prevent pregnancy.

consciousness: the patient is awake or is asleep but can be woken.

constipation: pain or difficulty passing *faeces*.

contraception: any method of delaying or preventing pregnancy.

convulsion: (also called a *fit*): the patient becomes stiff and may shake. The patient cannot stop the stiffness or control the shaking.

counselling: to help the patient to decide what to do.

dehydration: the result of loss of a large amount of water and salts from the body, usually caused by diarrhoea.

disease: an illness or group of illnesses. Very severe febrile disease is a group of diseases that includes several severe illnesses.

dysentery: diarrhoea with blood in the *faeces*.

examine: to look at, listen to, or feel, parts of the body to find out what is wrong.

faeces: stool. The waste that comes out of the end of the *bowel*.

fallopian tubes: the tubes through which eggs pass to reach the inside of the *uterus*.

family planning: to use methods to delay or to prevent pregnancy. To have the number of children that a family wants, when the family wants the children.

febrile: to have a *fever*.

fever: when the body temperature is high. This may mean: that the patient or mother tells you that the patient had a fever; the patient feels hot to touch; the temperature under the arm is 37.5°C (99.5°F) or higher, or in the *rectum* or mouth is 38°C (100.4°F) or higher.

fit: see *convulsion*.

folic acid: folic acid or folate, is a *vitamin* found in food that the body needs to help it make red blood cells.

foreign body: a thing which is not part of the human body, for example a stone in the ear.

fungus: germs that grow like moulds and which can cause *infections*. Anti-fungal treatments fight fungus infections.

generic: the normal name of a medicine. Generic medicines are cheaper than brand name medicines.

haemoglobin: a red protein that contains iron. Haemoglobin carries *oxygen*.

hookworm: hookworm are small *parasites* which live in a person's intestine and suck blood.

hygiene: clean habits which prevent *disease*. This includes preparing food in a clean way, drinking water from a protected water source, putting *faeces* in latrines or covered holes, washing regularly.

hypoglycaemia: low blood sugar.

immune system: the system that helps the body to fight *disease*. The immune system makes *antibodies* or special cells to fight disease.

immunisation: a medicine which will protect against a *disease*. Also called *vaccines*. Some immunisations are injected and some are drunk. There are immunisations for tuberculosis, tetanus, polio, diphtheria, measles, mumps and rubella. Other immunisations may be available in some countries.

infection: an illness caused by *bacteria*, *viruses* or other very small living things.

intramuscular (IM) injection: an injection put into a muscle, usually into the upper leg.

intravenous (IV) injection: an injection put into a vein.

jaundice: a yellow colour in the white part of the eyes and the skin.

joints: places where bones meet.

Kernig's sign: a pain felt in the back, neck or head when the patient's hip is bent and the knee straightened. It is used to diagnose *meningitis*.

kidneys: two organs behind the *abdomen* which make *urine* by cleaning waste from the blood.

loss of consciousness: see *unconscious*.

lymph nodes: small lumps under the skin which trap and fight *infections*. Lymph nodes become swollen and often painful if they become infected.

mastoid: the part of the skull bone behind the ear.

measles complications: problems or *infections* that occur during or after measles. Diarrhoea, pneumonia and skin infections are examples of measles complications.

meningitis: meningitis is an infection of the outside of the brain. Meningitis is caused either by *bacteria* or *viruses*.

menstrual period: bloody fluid which leaves a woman's *uterus*, passes through the *vagina* and out of the private parts. This happens about every 28 days and lasts for a few days.

microscope: an instrument that makes very small things look larger.

minerals: simple substances in foods that help to build the body and help the body fight *disease*. Iron is an example of a mineral.

nausea: the patient feels as if he may vomit.

nipple: the middle of the round, dark part of the breast. In women, this is where milk for the baby comes out.

nutrition: the food people eat. Good nutrition is important: it means eating a mixed diet to help the body to grow and fight disease.

oral rehydration solution: a solution made with oral rehydration salts (ORS), a mixture of glucose and salts: sodium chloride 3.5 g/l; trisodium citrate 2.9 g/l, potassium chloride 1.5 g/l; and glucose 20.0 g/l.

oxygen: a gas in air that the body needs to live.

parasite: very small worms and animals that can live inside people and cause *disease*, for example malaria and schistosomiasis.

period: a short way of referring to *menstrual period*.

prescriber: a trained health worker who decides what medicines to give to patients.

private parts: the parts of the bodies of men and women which allow people to have *sexual intercourse* to produce babies. These parts include the woman's *vagina* and the man's penis.

pulse: the movement of an artery each time the heart beats. The pulse rate tells you how many times the heart beats in one minute.

pus: yellow or green fluid in wounds or *abscesses* caused by the body fighting *infection*.

rectum: the lower part of the *bowel*. *Faeces* are stored in the rectum.

refer: to send a patient to be seen by another health worker.

respiratory distress: a patient with respiratory distress finds it very difficult to breathe.

schistosomiasis: a *parasite* that enters the body through the skin.

scrotum: the bag between a man's legs that holds his testes (testicles).

sexual intercourse: sex with the penis in the *vagina*.

shock: a dangerous problem which results in not enough blood reaching the brain and other parts of the body.

sign: something that you see, hear or feel which helps you decide which *disease* the patient has, for example fast breathing or *chest indrawing*.

sterilise: to kill *bacteria*, *viruses* and *fungus* on a piece of equipment, usually by steaming or boiling it for 20 minutes. At high altitudes, the steaming or boiling time must be much longer.

stethoscope: an instrument used to listen to sounds inside the body.

subcutaneous injection: an injection given under the skin.

symptom: something the patient tells you about, or which you can see, which helps you to decide which *disease* the patient has.

syringe: an instrument used to inject medicine.

temperature: see *fever*.

tutorial: a lesson between a trainer and one student or a few students.

ulcer: a painful open sore.

unconscious: a state in which an ill or injured patient seems to be asleep but cannot be awakened.

ureter: tubes in the *abdomen* which carry *urine* from the *kidneys* to the *bladder*.

urine: fluid waste that collects in the *bladder*.

uterus: also called the womb. Where the baby grows inside a pregnant woman.

vaccinations or vaccines: an injection or medicine to drink which will protect against a *disease*.

vagina: a tube of muscle from the entrance of the *uterus* (called *cervix*) to the opening between a woman's legs. This is where a baby passes when it is born.

vein: a tube which carries blood towards the heart. There is no *pulse* when you touch a vein.

virus: a very tiny germ that causes *infections*. *Antibiotics* do *not* fight viruses.

vitamins: parts of food that help to build the body and help the body to fight *disease*. Vitamin C, vitamin A and folic acid are examples of vitamins.

List of useful resources for health workers

Anaemia in Rural Africa. Community support for control activities where malaria is common. Elizabeth Topley. FSG MediMedia Ltd and DFID 1998.

Clinical Tuberculosis, Second edition. John Crofton, Norman Horne, Fred Miller. Macmillan 1999.

Diseases of Children in the Subtropics and Tropics, Fourth edition. Edited by Paget Stanfield, Martin Brueton, Michael Chan, Michael Parkin, Tony Waterstone. Educational Low-Priced Books with Edward Arnold 1991.

Essential Drugs, slide set. available from TALC, PO Box 49, St Albans, Hertfordshire, AL1 5TX, UK.

Helping Health Workers Learn. A book of methods, aids and ideas for instructors at the village level. David Werner and Bill Bower. The Hesperian Foundation 1982.

Integrated Management of Childhood Illness. World Health Organization and UNICEF 1997.

The Management of Acute Respiratory Infections in Children: Practical guidelines for outpatients care. World Health Organization 1995.

Management of Severe and Complicated Malaria – A practical handbook. World Health Organization 1991.

Manson's Topical Diseases, Twentieth edition. Edited by Gordon Cook. Educational Low-Priced Books with W.B. Saunders 1996.

Natural Medicine in the Tropics. Dr Hans Martin-Hirt and Bindanda M'Pia, 1995. Available from Anamed, Schafweide 77, D-71364 Winneden, Germany.

Oxford Handbook of Clincal Medicine, Fourth edition. R.A. Hope, J.M. Longmore, S.K. McManus, C.A. Wood-Allum. Oxford University Press 1998.

Oxford Handbook of Clinical Specialities, Fourth edition. J.A.B. Collier, J.M. Longmore, T.J. Hodgetts. Oxford University Press 1994.

Practical General Practice. Guidelines for effective clinical management, Third edition. Alex Khot and Andrew Polmear. Butterworth Heinemann 1999.

Where Women Have No Doctor. A health guide for women. A. August Burns, Ronnie Lovich, Jane Maxwell, Katherine Shapiro. Macmillan 1997.

Other references used in writing this manual

Unaumwa na nini? Mafunzo ya afya ya msingi. (What is your problem? Lessons in primary health care.) Keith Birrell and Ginny Birrell. Ministry of Health, Zanzibar, Tanzania 1996.

The Use of Essential Drugs. Sixth report of the WHO Expert Committee. WHO Technical Report Series No. 850. World Health Organization 1995.

Guidelines for the Use of Iron Supplements to Prevent and Treat Iron Deficiency Anemia. Rebecca J. Stolzfus, Michele L. Dreyfuss. International Nutritional Anemia Consultative Group, World Health Organization, United Nations Children's Fund, International Life Sciences Institute Press 1998.

British National Formulary. Number 37. British Medical Association and Royal Pharmaceutical Society of Great Britain 1999.

VSO Books

VSO Books is the publishing unit of VSO. Since 1958, more than 27,000 skilled volunteers have worked alongside national colleagues in over 60 countries throughout the developing world. VSO Books publishes practical books and Working Papers in education and development based upon current thinking and professional experience of volunteers and their overseas partners. Working Papers in Development are published for free downloading on VSO's web site www.vso.org.uk/pubs/wpapers/

VSO Books Titles Include:

Books for development workers

Adult Literacy – A handbook for development workers, Paul Fordham, Deryn Holland, Juliet Millican, VSO/Oxfam Publications, 192pp, ISBN 0 85598 315 9

Care and Safe Use of Hospital Equipment, Muriel Skeet, David Fear, VSO Books, 188pp, ISBN 0 9509050 5 4

Culture, Cash and Housing – Community and tradition in low-income housing, Andy Bevan, Maurice Mitchell, VSO/ITP, 128pp, ISBN 1 85339 153 0

How to Grow a Balanced Diet, Ann Burgess, Grace Maina, Philip Harris, Stephanie Harris, VSO Books, 244pp, ISBN 0 9509050 6 2

Made in Africa – Learning from carpentry hand-tool projects, Janet Leek, Andrew Scott, Matthew Taylor, VSO/ITP, 70pp, ISBN 1 85339 214 6

Managing for a Change – How to run community development projects, Anthony Davies, ITP, 160pp, ISBN 1 85339 339 1

Water Supplies for Rural Communities, Colin and Mog Ball, VSO/ITP, 56pp, ISBN 1 85339 112 3

Books for teachers

The Agricultural Science Teachers' Handbook, Peter Taylor, VSO Books, 148pp, ISBN 0 9509050 7 0

The English Language Teacher's Handbook, Joanna Baker/Heather Westrup, VSO/Continuum, 170pp, ISBN 0 304 70642 6

The Handbook for Teaching Sports, National Coaching Foundation, VSO/Heinemann, 160pp, ISBN 0 435 92320 X

How to Make and Use Visual Aids, Nicola Harford, Nicola Baird, VSO/Heinemann, 128pp, ISBN 0 435 92317 X

Introductory Technology – A resource book, Adrian Owens, VSO/ITP, 142pp, ISBN 1 85339 064X

The Maths Teachers' Handbook, Jane Portman, Jeremy Richardson, VSO/Heinemann, 108pp, ISBN 0 435 92318 8

Participatory Forestry – The process of change in India and Nepal, Mary Hobley, 338pp, VSO/ODI, ISBN 0 85003 204 0

The Science Teachers' Handbook, Andy Byers, Ann Childs, Chris Lainé, VSO/ Heinemann, 144pp, ISBN 0 435 92302 1

Setting Up and Running a School Library, Nicola Baird, VSO/Heinemann, 144pp, ISBN 0 435 2304 8 4

For more information about VSO Books, contact: VSO Books, 317 Putney Bridge Road, London SW15 2PN, UK. Tel: +44 208 780 7200, fax: +44 208 780 7300. web site: www.vso.org.uk. email: silke.bernau@vso.org.uk

VSO is the largest independent volunteer-sending agency in the world.

VSO health professionals work in all areas of assessment, prevention, education outreach and primary health care for the disadvantaged. If you have a background in any health-related field and 2 years experience and want to find out more about how to become a VSO volunteer, contact VSO Enquiries Unit, 317 Putney Bridge Road, London SW15 2PN, UK. Tel: +44 208 780 7500, fax: +44 208 780 7300, email: enquiry@vso.org.uk. web site: www.vso.org.uk

If you would like to request a VSO volunteer, in health or any other professional area, please contact the VSO programme office in your country, who will be pleased to discuss your needs.

Index

Note: Numbers in **bold** show pictures;
numbers in *italics* show tables.
<u>Underlined</u> numbers show an
important entry.

abdomen, areas of the **106**, **109**, 110–20
abdominal problems 104–23
  abdominal pain 9, 87, 96, 98, 100,
    102, <u>104–5</u>, 166, <u>226</u>, 227, 231,
    <u>232</u>
      constant <u>105</u>, *107*, **107**, *112*, *113*,
        114, 117, 121, 122
      intermittent <u>105</u>, *106*, **107**, *112*,
        113, 115, 118, 119, 120, 122
    bleeding inside 98
    common and important abdominal
      problems 110–11, *112*, *113*,
      114–21
    how to examine the abdomen
      108–10, **109**
    how to take an abdominal history
      <u>108</u>, 123
abortion, threatened abortion 98, 227
abscess 73, <u>74–5</u>
    breast <u>75</u>, 84
    caused by injections 21
    tooth 180, <u>184</u>, *185*, <u>234</u>, 249, 251
    treatment <u>75</u>, *80*, 84
    tuberculosis <u>161</u>, 162
acetylsalicylic acid *see* aspirin
acid fast bacilli (AFBs) 32, <u>162</u>, <u>165</u>
acute dacrocystitis *see* dacrocystitis,
    acute
acute glaucoma *see under* glaucoma
adrenaline *see* epinephrine
AIDS (Acquired ImmunoDeficiency
    Syndrome) 170, <u>171</u>, 173
albendazole 245
alcohol
    intoxication 149–50
    withdrawal 149–50
allergy 78–9, *82*, 137, 192, 196
aluminium hydroxide 102–3, 114, 245
alveoli **26**, 27
aminophylline 34, *35*, 245
amoxicillin 31, 32, *32*, 97, 102, 120,
    173, 180, 227, 232, 234, 246
ampicillin 102
anaemia 10, 29, 30, <u>59</u>, 108, 156, 165,
    180, 191, 213, 232
    and blood pressure 131
    causes 59
    diagnosing 62
    and heavy periods 59, *63*, 69, 96
    moderate 62
    in pregnancy 59, 62, *63*, 64, 65–6, <u>99</u>
    preventing 60–2
    severe 48, <u>62</u>, 125
    and sickle cell disease 217–18
    treatment 51, 62, *63*, 64, *64*, <u>212</u>, 248
anaphylaxis *82*, **136**, <u>137</u>, 144, 208, 248
angina 125, <u>126</u>, <u>127</u>, *129*
antepartum haemorrhage (APH) 98,
    227
antibiotics
    and anaphylaxis 137
    bought from a shopkeeper 15, 16
    injections 208

side effects <u>16</u>, 78
    for sinusitis 173
    treating infections caused by
      bacteria 16
antibody test 172
anxiety 27, 98, 126, 135, 148, 149,
    <u>152</u>, <u>154–5</u>, 156, 159
appendicitis 86, *106*, *107*, <u>111</u>, *112*,
    <u>114</u>, 122, 232
arteries 127
arthritis 141–2
    osteoarthritis 142, 251
    rheumatoid arthritis 142, 251
    septic <u>142</u>, 144, 162, 217, 247
aspirin (acetylsalicylic acid) 18, 114,
    122, 127, *129*, 131, 245
asthma <u>27</u>, 30–7
atenolol 129

back pain *106*, 111, <u>142–4</u>, 162, 167,
    <u>233</u>
bacteria
    antibiotics 16, 21
    bottle-feeding *55*, 91
    chest illnesses 27
    corneal ulcers 193
    food poisoning 86
    skin infections 73–6, *80*
    tonsillitis 181–2, **182**, 183
    urinary tract infection 119
bananas 129
bendroflumethiazide (bendrofluazide)
    129
benzathine penicillin 125
benzyl benzoate emulsion 21, 77, <u>78</u>,
    81, 246
benzylpenicillin 8–9, 28–31, *33*, 34,
    42, 50, *80*, 82, 98, 102, 180, 183,
    185, 193–4, 197, 218, 227, 234–5,
    248, 251, 253
betamethasone 180
Bitot's spots **199**, 200, 252
bleeding
    after sexual intercourse 96, 97, 226
    from the nose 186–7, *186*
    from the vagina 96–7, 226
    from the vagina after birth 101,
      208, 227, 248
    from the vagina before birth 98,
      100, 227
    inside the abdomen 98
    into the bowel 61
blindness/poor sight 127, 163, 165,
    <u>189</u>, 191, 197, 229
blisters 72, 163, 167
blood
    blood loss and shock 136, 144
    cough with 27, 162, 167, 176
    in the faeces 9, 10, <u>87</u>, 89, 91, 115,
      119, 232
    in the urine 119–20
blood cells
    damage to red 59, 61
    red 59, 61, 217, 231
    white 74, 170–1, 231
blood pressure 127, 191, 235
    and age 128
    diastolic 99, 127, 128, 130
    examination for 128–31, **130**
    high 99, 100, 125, 127–9, *129*, 187
    in pregnancy <u>99–100</u>, 128, 129, *129*,
      131
    systolic 127, 130

blood sugar
    low <u>46</u>, 213, 230
    preventing low 8, 24, 47, 50
blood transfusion 99, 171, 174, 213,
    218
blood vessel damage 99
body, illness of 148, 149–50
body lice 77, *81*
bones
    broken 134–5, **135**, 136, **136**, 144,
      233, 247
    infection of 142
    tuberculosis of 162, 233
bottle, for measuring liquid medicine
    211
bottle-feeding 55, 91, 94, 171
botulin toxin 225
bowel, blocked 105
brain damage 99, 157
brand name medicine 20, 22
breast abscess *see* abscess
breastfeeding 18, 94
    breastmilk substitute 8
    a child with malnutrition 214
    delays the next pregnancy 62
    diet while 52
    duration of (2 years) 5, 54, 69, 91
    expressed breastmilk 8, 50, 75, *80*,
      84, 214
    HIV-infected mother 171
    insufficient breastmilk *54*
    preventing anaemia 61
    and soft foods 54, *55*, 69, 91
    unable to breastfeed 7, 47, 89, 91
    vitamin A in breastmilk 200
    while pregnant *55*, 65
breathing
    difficulty 10, 33, 35, 72, 225
    treating children 206, 207
    fast 20, <u>29</u>, *29*, **31**, 33–6, 59, 62,
      64, 72, 125, *129*, 154, 218, 232
broken bones *see* bones
bronchi **26**, 27, 161
bronchitis 27, 32, 246–7
bronchodilators 29, 31, 34, *35*
brushing/cleaning teeth *see* teeth
burns 138–41
    degree of 139, 144
    and leprosy 165

candida, oral 172–3, 176, 184, *185*,
    229, 249
carbamazepine 152, 157
carbohydrate 52, *53*, 230
cassava, bitter cassava poisoning 225
Cassia alata 219, **219**
cataract 189, 200–1, **200**, 236
cellulitis <u>73</u>, 74, *80*, 84, 180, 234, 246,
    247, 251
    orbital <u>202</u>, 236
cerebral malaria *see* malaria
cerebrovascular incident (CVI) <u>127</u>, 229
cervix 100
chest illnesses 25–37, 71
    in an adult or a child aged 6 years
      or more 30–2
    in children aged 5 years or less
      27–30
    home treatment 35
    how to treat wheeze 33–4, *35*, 245
    when to send patients to hospital 36
chest indrawing <u>28</u>, **28**, 30, 31, 33
chest pain 217

chest X-ray 162, 168
chickenpox 72, *79*, 84
children
  anaemia 59, 213
  burns and skin area 140–1, **140**
  chest illness (aged 5 years or less) 27–30
  chest illness (aged 6 years or more) 30–32
  cough or difficult breathing 206, 207
  diarrhoea in 85
  eating a mixed diet 52
  fast breathing *29*
  feeding 60, <u>54</u>, 75, 88, 91
  with severe malnutrition 214–15
  growth chart *see* growth chart
  and HIV 171, 176, 178
  malnutrition danger times 54, *54–5*
  preventing malaria 61
  preventing malnutrition 53
  and rectal prolapse 121
  serious skin infections in children less than 2 months old 76, *81*, 82
  severe malnutrition *see* malnutrition
  sickle cell disease 217–18
  and six rules of good nutrition 54
  tuberculosis 162
  vaccinations 11
  weighing 57, 213
chlamydia 197
chloramphenicol 8, 24, 28, 30–1, 50, 76, *81*, 82, 94, 102, 180, 183, *185*, 234, 246, 248
chloroquine 8, 18, 24, 29, 38, 39, <u>42–5</u>, 49, *63*, 94, 101, 247, 252
chloroquine-resistant malaria *see* malaria
chlorpromazine 151
cholera <u>87</u>, 88–9, 92, 253
cholera treatment centre 94
chronic glaucoma *see under* glaucoma
clofazimine 165–6
co-trimoxazole 16, 17, 20, 29, 31–2, *33*, 42, 73–6, *80*, 84, <u>88</u>, *88*, 117, 139, 142, 173, 180, *185*, 211, 218, 234, 247
coconut oil 79, *82*, 188
coconut water 91, 222, **223**
coma position 133, **133**
communication 12–13
condoms 169, 171, 174, 177, 178
congenital heart disease 125
conjunctiva 62, 189, 198, 218, 228
conjunctivitis 17, 71
  allergic 196–7, **196**, 235
  bacterial 196, 235, 253
  chlamydial 197–8, 235, 253
  gonococcal 197, 235, 251, 253
  viral 18, 195–6, **195**, 197, 235
consciousness, loss of 98, 100, 134, 137, 144
constipation *106*, *113*, 118, <u>119</u>
contraceptive pill <u>96</u>, 102, 226, 247
convulsions 7–10, 24, 228, 247–8
  and alcohol withdrawal 149
  causes <u>46</u>, <u>47</u>
  and epilepsy 156, *158*
  febrile 46, 49, 156
  and head injury 156
  in meningitis 47, 48
  in pregnancy 99, 100, 249
  prevention 18–19, 46

cord, prolapsed umbilical cord 100, 228
cornea 42, <u>190</u>, 191, 192, 194–5, 197, 235–6
corneal abrasion 195, 235
corneal scar 197, 201, **201**, 236
corneal ulcer 71, *79*, 165, 192–3, **193**, 235, 252–3
coronary arteries 126
cough 10, 15, 16, *26*, <u>27</u>, 30, 71
  with blood 27, 162, 167–8, 176
  in measles 71, 87
  pain in ribs 27, 31
  with sputum 176
  treating children aged 5 years or less 206–7
  in tuberculosis 160, 162, 167
counselling 153, <u>154</u>, 156, 172
  about HIV testing 175–6
cross-eyes 199, **199**, 236
cryptococcus 172–3
cup and spoon, for feeding children *see* children
cutaneous leishmaniasis 74, 83

dacrocystitis, acute <u>202–3</u>, **202**, 236, 247, 251
dapsone 165–6, 168
degree (of burn) *see* burns
dehydration 85, 87–90, 93, 139, 221–2, 250
deltamethrin 218
delusions <u>148</u>, 151–2
depression 148, <u>152–3</u>, 156, *158*, 159
diabetes 46, 73–4, 83, 119, 156, 161, 191, <u>229–30</u>
diabetic ketoacidosis 229, 230
diarrhoea 10, 85–94
  and bottle-feeding *55*
  causes 86, 94
  dehydration 85, 87–90, 93
  and milk 215
  preventing 90–91
  a side-effect of antibiotics 16
  taking a history and examination 86–7
  treatment 88–90, 91, 220, 222, **223**
diastolic blood pressure 99, 127–8, 130
diazepam 8, 100, 135–6, 146, 149, 154, 228, 247
  giving rectally 210, **210**
diet, mixed 16, 18, 24, 32, 50, <u>52</u>, <u>53</u>, *55*, 57, 59, 61, *63*, 66, 71, 73, *79*, 91, 99, 121, 172, 173, 184, 216, 229, 234, 248
diphtheria 181–2, **182**, 183, *185*
direct recording scale 51, 55, 67–8
Directly Observed Treatment (DOT) programmes 162
disc prolapse 143–4, 145
discharge
  from the ear 180, *185*, <u>234</u>
  from the penis 117
  from the vagina 96, 102, 174, <u>226</u>
dressings
  for burns 138
  for wounds 134
drink
  clean water 16
  unable to 7, 8, 10, 35, 72, 89, 91, 181, 183
dysentery <u>87</u>, <u>88</u>, *88*, 89, 247, 250
dystonia, acute 151, *158*

ear
  discharge from 180, *185*, 234
  foreign body in 180, *185*, 187–8
  infection 30, 32, 180, 234
  itching in 180, 234
  noises in 180, 234
  swelling near to 180, 234
  swelling of 180
  treating an ear problem 234
  wax blocking 188
early pregnancy 97–8, 227
  see also pregnancy, vomiting in
eating, unable to eat 10, 33, 37, 183
eclampsia 99, 249
ectopic pregnancy 97, <u>98</u>, *107*, *112*, <u>117</u>, 226–7, 232
eczema 78, <u>79</u>, *82*
education, importance in preventing malnutrition 216
energy 52, *53*, 55
ENL reaction 166
epiglottitis 28, 30, <u>181</u>, *183*, *185*, 246
epilepsy 46, 148, <u>156–7</u>, *158*
epinephrine 34, *35*, 137, *137*, 144, 208, 248
ergometrine 208, 248
erythromycin 197, 248, 253
ethambutol 162–3
examination 10
exercise 27, 127–8, 131, 143–4, 163, 229–30, 233
eyelids 189, 190–91, **191**, 194
eyes
  anaemia signs 62, 64–5
  corneas 42
  cross- 199, **199**, 236
  examining 190–1
  foreign body in 194–5, 235
  front of a normal eye 189–90, **190**
  irritation of 235
  pain in 16, 191–4
  red eye 192–8, 235, 236, 251
  symptoms and signs 192
eyesight, problems with 198–203, 229, 235–6, 251

faeces
  blood in 9, 10, 87, 89, 91, 115, 119, <u>232</u>
  and hygiene 91
fallopian tubes, infection 117
Fansidar 29, 38, 40, <u>42</u>, 43, <u>44</u>, 45–6, 49, *63*, 101–3, 248, 250, 252
febrile convulsions 46, 49
feeding children *see* children
feeling, unusual feeling in arms/legs 134, 146, 165, 168
feeling, lack of, in skin 164, 168
ferrous sulphate 51, 62, *63*, 64, <u>64</u>, 66, 99, 102–3, 213, 218, 248
fever
  sending a patient to hospital 48
  treatment for 8, 17–19, <u>40–42</u>
filarial worms 116
fits *see* convulsions
flea bites 73, 77, *81*
fluphenazine 151
folic acid 51, 52, *53*, <u>59–62</u>, 99, 102, 103, 213, 218, 248
food poisoning <u>86</u>, *106*, *113*, 119, 225, 232
foods
  allergy 137

foods (*Contd*)
  hygiene 16, 91, 92
  nutritious 52, *53*
  soft 54, *55*, 69, 91
  to prevent anaemia 60–1
foreign body
  in the ear 180, *185*, 187–8
  in the eye 194–5, 235
  in the nose *186*, 187
fruit 53–4, 61, 91, 119, 172, 200
fungus infections 70, 76–7, *81*, 165,
    193, 246
  making treatments 219
furosemide 213

gangrene 229
gastritis *107*, *112*, 114, 245
gastroenteritis 24, 86, 93, *106*, *113*,
    119, 232
general danger signs 7–8
generic medicine 20, 22
gentian violet 21, 73, 77, *80*, *81*, 138,
    184, *185*, 248
gingivitis 184
glasses 198, 204, 236
glaucoma
  acute 194, **194**, 235
  chronic 201–2, 236
gonococcal conjunctivitis 197–8
gonorrhoea 197
good nutrition *see* nutrition
grass pea poisoning 225
growth chart 11, 19, 51, 55–7, 64–6,
    67, 68, **68**, 93
guarding 110, 111, 122, 232, 245
gums 184
gynaecology clinic 97, 226
gynaecology problems 95–7

haemoglobin 52, 59–62, 64, 66, 99,
    213, 228
hair, and malnutrition 57
hairy leucoplakia, oral 171, 173, 176
hallucinations 148–52
haloperidol 151
head injury 133–4, 144
  and convulsions 156, *158*
  and severe mental illness 149–50
headache 65, 99, 118, 128, 134,
    154–5, 173, 176, 224
health centres
  safe procedures in 174, 178
  tutorials 237–44
healthy heart advice 128–9
hearing, poor 180, 234
heart beat, patient aware of 128, 131,
    154, 155
heart failure 125, **125**, 127, *129*, 162
  how to look for 131
heart, how to examine 125
hepatitis 21, *107*, *113*, 120–21
hernia 115–16, **115**
  incarcerated *106*, *107*, *112*, 116, 232
herpes zoster 171, *172*, 176, 193
history, how to take a patient's history
    7–11
  general danger signs 7–8
  taking a history 9–11
hookworm 59, 61, *63*, 66, 99, 228,
    245, 248, 249
Human Immunodeficiency Virus
    (HIV) 21, 161, 164, 169–78, 215
hydrocoele 115–16, **116**
hydrocortisone 79, *82*

hygiene 16, 86, 91, 92
hypertension *see* blood pressure, high
hypoglycaemia *see* blood sugar, low

ibuprofen 20, 96, 114, 120, 122, 142,
    173, 226, 249
illness of the body *see* body
immune system 161, 172
impetigo 72–3, 77–8, *80*, *81*, 247,
    249–51
infections
  and anaemia *63*
  avoiding 16
  bacterial *see* bacterial infections
  of the bone 142
  and burns 139
  fungus *see* fungus infections
  and HIV 171
  of a joint 142
  of the kidney *107*, *113*, 120
  skin 73–6, 229
  upper respiratory 16, 24, 27, 30, 41
  of the urinary tract 97–8, 102–3,
    107, *113*, 119–20
  yeast 77, *81*, 84, 219, 229
  see also meibomian cyst
inhalers 25, 34, **34**
injections
  causing abscesses 21
  giving 208–9, **209**
insects 77–8
  bites/stings 73, 77, *81*, 137
insulin 46, 229, 230
intussusception 86, *106*, *112*, 114–15,
    115, 232
iodine 138, 177
  polyvidone 74, 75, *80*, 84, 134, 138,
    169, 252
iris 190–1
iritis 192–3, **193**, 204
iron 52, 53, 59, 60–2
irritation, of the eyes 235
isoniazid 162
itching
  in the ear 180, 234
  in the private parts 231
ivermectin 78, 202

jaundice 48, *108*, 120–1, 163, 167, 232
joints
  painful 141, 217
  swollen 141

kala azar 45–6
Kaposi's sarcoma 172, 173, 176
Kernig's sign 38, 48
kerosene poisoning *138*, 144
ketoacidosis 229–30
kidneys
  damage 99, 229
  failure 127
  infection *107*, *113*, 120, 246
  kidney stones *106*, *113*, 120, 231, 249
  painful 110
kwashiorkor 58, **58**, 66–7

labour *106*, 110–11, *112*, 227, 232
latrines 61, *63*, 91, 92, 231
lens 190, 200–1
leprosy 164–7
  borderline 164–6, 168
  and fungus infections 76, 83
  lepromatous 164–6, 168
  and skin ulcers 73

tuberculoid 164–5
lidocaine hydrochloride 249
light reflection test 199, 236
light-headedness 186, 230
liver, large 110
lymph nodes 161–2, 167

magnesium sulphate 100, 103, 228, 249
malaria 8, 10, 41, 118, 213, 247
  cerebral 24, 46, 47, 149–50
  chloroquine-resistant 44–5, 49
  damages red blood cells 59, 61
  diagnosis and management 39–40
  diarrhoea in 49, 86, 94
  Fansidar-resistant 38, 44, 45–6, 49
  fever in 87, 143
  prevention 61, 63, 218
  and sickle cell disease 217
malnutrition 165
  causes of 52
  danger times for children 54, 54–5
  early 55, 57, 65
  prevention 52–3, 88, 89
  severe 55, 57–9, **58**, 68, 87
    examination and diagnosis 213
    feeding 214
    recipes 215
    treatment 213–14, 252
  the six rules of good nutrition 54
  treatment 57, 58–9, 88, 212
  see also kwashiorkor
mania 149, 151–2
marasmus *see* malnutrition
mastoiditis 180, 234, 246, 251
Maternal and Child Health clinic 57,
    96–7, 99
measles **16**, 17, 42, 71–2, 79, 82, 196,
    235, 252
  diagnosing 71
  diarrhoea in 86
  and pneumonia 79, 82
measuring bottle, for liquid medicines
    211
mebendazole 57, *63*, 65, 99, 214, 228,
    231, 249
medicines
  antipsychotic 151–2
  bought from a shop 15–16
  for high blood pressure 127, 129
  and jaundice 120, 163, 167
  leprosy 165–6
  list of medicines and their uses
    245–53
  a measuring bottle for liquid
    medicines 211
  not to be used in pregnancy 98, 102
  reaction to 78, 79, *82*
  safe to use in pregnancy or while
    breastfeeding 101–2
  side effects of 16
  taking correctly 22–3
  to cure illness (disease) 18, 22
  to prevent pregnancy 96, 102, 226,
    247
  to treat symptoms 18, 22
meibomian cyst, infected 203, **203**, 236
meningitis 8, 24, 41, 46, 47
  and severe mental illness 149–50
  signs of meningitis in patients aged
    more than 6 months 48, 50
  signs of meningitis in patients aged
    under 6 months 47–8, 50
meningococcal septicaemia 73, *80*, 82

mental illness, severe 148–52, *158*
metronidazole 184, *185*, 234, 249
milk 8, 24, 50, 114, 149, 213, 221
   nutrition 214–15
minerals 52, *55*, 69
mixed diet, importance of 16, 18, 24,
   32, 50, <u>52</u>, <u>53</u>, *55*, 57, 59, 61, *63*,
   66, 71, 73, *79*, 91, 99, 121, 172–3,
   184, *216*, *229*, 234, 248
methylrosanilinium chloride 249
mosquito nets 61, 218
mother, teaching the 216
mouth
   pain in 16, 184
   ulcers 57, 184
multivitamins 249–50
mumps 173, <u>180</u>, 234
muscles
   and malnutrition 57, 58
   and polio 224
mycobacteria <u>161</u>, 162, <u>164</u>, 165–6
Mycobacterium leprae 164
Mycobacterium tuberculosis 161
myocardial infarction (MI) 125,
   <u>126–7</u>, *129*, 229

nalidixic acid 250
nasogastric tube 8, 88, 90, 93–4, 214,
   225, 230
   how to put in a <u>221</u>
nausea 16, 126, 154–5
nephritis 231
nerve damage 164, 167–8, 229
night blindness <u>200</u>, 236, 252
noises in the ear *see* tinnitus
non-typhi salmonella 172, <u>173</u>
normal saline 73–5, 134, 138, 250, 252
nose
   bleeds *see* bleeding
   foreign body in *186*, 187
nutrition
   good 52–3
   six rules of <u>53–4</u>, 57, 65, 213, 216,
     224, 236
nutrition clinic 58–9, <u>213–16</u>
nutrition milk 214–15
nutrition porridge 214–16
nystatin 184

obstetric problems 97–102, 227–8
onchocerciasis 78, 201, 236
operation scars 108
oral contraceptive pill <u>96</u>, 102, 226, 247
oral rehydration salts 88, <u>89</u>, <u>90</u>, 93,
   94, 98, 100–2, 117, 136, 173, 186,
   218, 221–2, 227, 230, 232, 250–51
orbital cellulitis <u>202</u>, 204, 236
orchitis 115, <u>117</u>, 247
osteoarthritis *see* arthritis
osteomyelitis <u>142</u>, 145, 217, 247
otitis externa <u>180</u>, 234, 246–7
otitis media 86–7, <u>180</u>, **234**, 246–7

pain
   in the abdomen 9, 87, 96–8, 100,
     102, <u>104–5</u>, *106–7*, **107**, 226–7,
     231–2
   in the back *106*, 111, <u>142–4</u>, 162,
     167, 233
   in the chest 31, 126, 217
   during sexual intercourse 96, <u>97</u>,
     102, 108, 175, 226, 232
   in the ear 180

every month when a woman has
     her period <u>96</u>, 108, 247, 249
   in the eye 16, <u>191–4</u>
   in the head 65, 99, 118, 128, 134,
     154–5, 173, 176, 224
   in a joint 141
   medicine to reduce 135
   in the mouth 184
   in the throat <u>180–3</u>, 224
   when coughing 27, 31
   while passing urine 102, 117, 119,
     122, 175
pale skin 165, 168
palpitations 228
paracetamol 17–18, 20, 41, 42, 46,
   102, 120, 142–4, 154, 166, 173,
   218, 224, 251
parotitis 172–3, 178, 180
pelvic inflammatory disease (PID) *107*,
   112, <u>117–18</u>, 232
penis, discharge from 117
peptic ulcer *107*, *112*, <u>114</u>, 122, 232, 245
pericarditis, tuberculous 125
periods 59, 96, 231
   and anaemia 59, *63*, 96
   painful 96, 108, 247, 249
   treatment 62, 226
peritoneum 111, 117
peritonitis 86, 92, 94, 98, *107*, <u>111</u>,
   114, 116–18, 232
   causes 111–19, 123
permethrin 61, 218
pethidine 135
phenobarbital 79, 157
phenoxymethylpenicillin 102, 183,
   185, 203, 251
phenytoin 157
pit latrines *see* latrines
placenta 101
pneumonia 8, 17, 20, 23, 25, <u>27</u>, <u>29</u>,
   30, <u>31</u>, *32*, 34–5, 41–2, 47, 62, *79*,
   171, 173, 176, 246, 247, 251
   diarrhoea in 86
   fever in 87, 125
   and measles *79*, 82
   pneumococcal 217
   Pneumocystitis carinii pneumonia
     (PCP) 171, 173
polio 92, 224–5
polyvidone iodine 74–5, *80*, 84, 134,
   169, 252
poor eyesight <u>189</u>, <u>198–203</u>, 229, 235,
   236, 251
porridge, nutrition 214–16
post-partum haemorrhage (PPH) <u>101</u>,
   208, 227, 248
poverty 53
pre-eclampsia 99
prednisolone 180
pregnancy
   age of first 62
   anaemia in 59, 62, *63*, 64–6, <u>99</u>
   blood pressure <u>99–100</u>, 128–9, *129*,
     131
   breastfeeding during *55*
   convulsions 99, 100
   diet in <u>52</u>, 53, *54*, 59
   ectopic 97, <u>98</u>, *107*, *112*, 117, 226–7,
     232
   frequency 59, 62, 69
   and HIV 171–2, 174, 178
   medicines not to be used during 98,
     102, 249

medicines safe to use during
     pregnancy 101–2
   preventing pregnancy <u>96</u>, 226, 247
   twin 98
   urinary tract infection 119–20
   vomiting in early pregnancy 97–8,
     227
prescribing *see* rational prescribing
private parts
   discharge from 96, 102, 174, 226
   itching in 231
   passing blood 98, 100–1
   ulcers near 102
procaine penicillin fortified 9, 21, 50,
   82, 94, 137, 180, 197, 234–5,
   248, 251, 253
prolapsed disc 143–4, 145
prolapsed rectum *113*, <u>121</u>, 232
prolapsed (umbilical) cord <u>100</u>, 228
protein 52, *53*, 54, *55*, 60, 99
psychiatric problems 120, 147–59
   anxiety <u>152–3</u>, 154–5, 156
   depression 152–3, 156
   epilepsy 156–7
   how to identify 155–6
   questions for psychiatric patients 148
   severe mental illness 148–52, 156
psychosis 148–9
pulmonary TB *see* tuberculosis
pulse 136–7, 186
pupil 190
pus <u>74</u>, 75–6, *81*, 139, 161, 174, 187,
   196–7
pyelonephritis *107*, *113*, <u>120</u>
pyrazinamide 162
pyrimethamine 42, 250

quinine 8, 18, 24, <u>45–6</u>, 94, 101, 103,
   252

rabies <u>138</u>, 144, 225
rashes
   chickenpox 72
   eczema 78, <u>79</u>, *82*
   fungus infections 76–7
   measles 16, **16**, 42, <u>71</u>, 196
   reaction to medicines <u>78</u>, 79, *82*,
     163, 167, 176
   a side-effect of medicines 16
rational prescribing 1, 15–25
rebound tenderness <u>110</u>, 111, 122,
   232, 245
rectal prolapse *113*, <u>121</u>, 232
relapsing fever 45, 46
respiratory distress 26, <u>33</u>, 36, 253
   signs of <u>33</u>, 37, 248
respiratory rate (speed of breathing)
   20, 24, <u>26–7</u>
retinol *see* vitamin A
reversal reaction 166
rheumatic heart disease 125
rheumatoid arthritis *see* arthritis
rifampicin 162–3, 165–6
river blindness 78
roundworm 245, 249
rupture, of the uterus <u>100–1</u>, 227

salbutamol <u>34</u>, **34**, <u>35</u>, 253
salt 129, 131
scabies 21, 70, 73, <u>78</u>, *81*, 246
schistosomiasis 120, 231
schizophrenia 149, <u>150–1</u>
scrotum, swellings in 115–16

septic arthritis *see* arthritis
septicaemia, meningococcal 73, *80*, **82**
sexual intercourse
  and HIV 174, 178
  and mental illness 152–3
  pain during 96, 97, 102, 108, 117,
    175, 226, 232
  passing blood after 96, 97, 226
  and TB patients 163, 166
  urinary tract infection 119
sexually-transmitted disease clinic 97,
  117, 197, 226, 232, 235
sexually-transmitted diseases 97, 102,
  103, 117, 171, 174–5, 176, 197,
  231
shingles *see* herpes zoster
shock 98, 136, 144, 186, 251
shoes 61, *63*, 167
sickle cell crisis 247, 251
sickle cell disease 59, 69, 217–18, 248
side effects, of medicines *see* medicines
signs
  of anaemia 62
  of diabetes 229
  of eye problems 192
  the four general danger signs 7–8
  of malnutrition in children 57–8
  of meningitis 47–8
  of respiratory distress 33
  of sickle cell disease 217
sinusitis 171, 173, 176, 217, 246, 247,
  253
six rules of good nutrition *see*
  nutrition
skin 70–84
  allergies 78–9
  bacterial infections 72–6, *80*
  burns and skin area 139, **140**, 141
  fluid under the skin 58, 62, 64, 131,
    215
  fungus infections 76–7, *81*, 246
  insects 77–8, *81*
  pale skin 165, 168
  rashes 16, 71–84, 176
  serious skin infections in children
    less than 2 months old 73, 76,
    81, 82
  swelling in the 165, 168
  treatment advice (leprosy patients)
    167
  ulcers 57, 70, 73–4, *80*, 83
  virus infections 71–2, *79–80*
skin-slit smear microscopy 165
sleeping sickness 148, 157, *158*
smoking 27, 96, 114, 122, 125, 126,
  128, 131, 230
snake bite 145–6
spacer 25, 34, 253
spine
  injury to 144, 145
  and tuberculosis 144, 145, 162, 168
spleen, large 61, *63*, 110
sputum 27, 30, 32, 176
sputum smear microscopy 162
sterilisation of needles and syringes
  174, 178, 209
steroid ear drops 180, 234
stethoscope 125, 130
Stevens-Johnson syndrome 163
stiff neck 41, 48
stones
  in a kidney 106, 113, 120, 231, 249

in a ureter 106, 113, 120
streptomycin 162, 163
stridor 28, 30, 31, 36, 181, 183
stroke 127
stye 203, **203**, 236
sub-conjunctival haemorrhage 198,
  198, 235
sugar water 8, 24, 50, 149, 213, 221
sugar–salt solution 91, 222, **223**
sulfadoxine 42
swelling
  abdominal 108, 232
  of the face *129*
  in a joint 141, 146
  of the legs 58, 62, 66, *129*, 141, 218,
    232
  of the liver *129*
  of a lymph node 162, 167
  near to the ear 180, 234
  near to the eye 58, 236
  of the neck *129*
  in the scrotum 115–16
  in the skin 165, 168
systolic blood pressure 127, 130

talk, unable to talk 33
teeth
  brushing/cleaning 184
  tooth abscess 180, 184, *185*, 234,
    249, 251
tepid sponging 8, 18–19, 24, 40, 41–2,
  46, 49, 50, *63*, 71, *79*
tetanus 21, 74, 134, 138
tetanus toxoid 84, 134, 138
tetracycline 17, 18, 42, 71, 173,
  193–7, 201, 203, 235, 251, 253
thioacetazone 162–3, 176
thioridazine 151
thirst 229
thoughts, disorganised/unusual 148,
  150–2
threadworms 231, 245, 249
throat **181**
  infection 30, 32, 180–83
  pain in 180–83, 188, 224
thrush 184
tick 225
tinea 76–7, *81*, 84
tinnitus 180
tiredness 156, 165, 228–9
tonsillitis 86, 181, 251
  bacterial 181–2, **182**, 183
  viral 181, **182**, 183
tooth *see* teeth
trachoma 196–7, **196**, 201, 235–6, 253
traditional healer 148, 152–3, 159
triamcinolone 180
trifluoperazine 151
trihexyphenidyl (benzhexol) 151, *158*
tuberculin skin testing *see* tuberculosis
tuberculoid leprosy *see* leprosy
tuberculosis (TB) 27, 32, 120, 160–3,
  171, 173, 215, 233
  extra-pulmonary 161
  pulmonary 161
  and the spine 144, 145, 162
  tuberculin skin testing for 162
tuberculous pericarditis *see* pericarditis
typhoid fever 45, 46, *107*, *112*, 118, 232

ulcers
  cleaning 73–4, 250, 252

corneal 71, *79*, 165, 192, 193, **193**,
  235, 252–3
  due to malnutrition 57
  and leprosy 165, 168
  in the mouth 57, 184
  near private parts 102, 174
  peptic *107*, *112*, 114, 122, 232, 245
  skin 57, 70, 73–4, *80*, 83
umbilical cord, prolapsed 100, 228
umbilicus, infection 76, *81*
unconsciousness 7, 133, 230, 248
upper respiratory infection 16, 24, 27,
  30, 41
ureters 105
  stones 106, 113, 120
urethra, irritation of 231
urinary tract infection 97–8, 102–3,
  107, *113*, 119–20, 122, 227, 231
urine
  blood in 119–20, 231
  and dehydration 87, 89
  frequent passing of 119, 229, 231
  interpreting results 231
  pain on passing 102, 117, 119, 122,
    175
  passing protein 99
  testing for sugar 191
urine microscopy 104, 120, 231
uterus
  infection 117
  rupture of the 100–101, 227

vaccinations 11, 74, 84, 134
vagina *see* private parts
vaseline 138, 187
vegetable fat 138
vegetable oil 119, 121, 188, 232
vegetables 53–4, 61, 91, 94, 119, 172,
  200
very severe febrile disease 8, 10, 24,
  31, 41, 46–8, 50, 88, 93, 150,
  156, *158*, 227, 230
viruses 16, 18, 27, 71–2, *79–80*, 138
  tonsillitis 181, **182**, 183
vitamin A (retinol) 17, 18, 42, 71,
  172, 189, 193–4, 196, 199–200,
  214, 235–6, 252
vitamin C 52, 53, 61
vitamins 52, 55
volvulus 106, 113, 118–19, 232
vomiting *see* pregnancy

warts 72, *80*
washing hands 16, 91, 119, 231
wax, in the ear 188
weakness, of an arm or leg 127, 165,
  168
weighing children 55, 57, 67, 213
weight loss 55, **56**, 57, 162, 167,
  172–3, 176, 215, 229
wheeze 27, 29–34, 206–7, 245, 253
whipworm 121, 245, 249
Whitfield ointment (benzoic acid and
  salicylic acid) 76, *81*, 84, 246, 253
worms 57, 116, 213–14
wounds
  cleaning 134, 138, 250, 252
  dressing of 134
  head 134
  treatment of 134, 249

yeast infections 77, *81*, 219, 229